ST3 Orthopaedic Interview Success: An essential guide for Orthopaedic interviews

Written by:

Manjunath.B.Ramappa

MBBS, MRCS, MSc, MCh, FHEA

Specialty Trainee in Trauma & Orthopaedics

Northern Deanery, UK

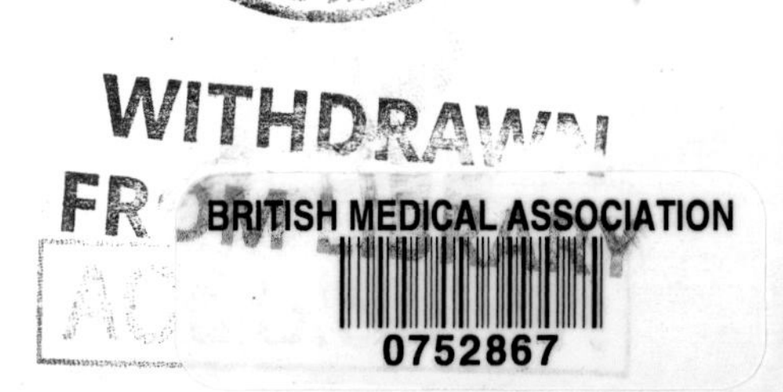

Published by Manjunath Limited
1st edition

ISBN 978-1-5262-0456-1

Printed July 2016

Printed in the United Kingdom by BookPrintingUK

The author has taken care to ensure accuracy of the information provided at the time of publication. Appropriate references are mentioned. This book should be used as an interview guide and is not intended for clinical management of patients.

Contents

Preface

This book aims to provide a thorough insight into orthopaedic interviews. Having been through the system myself, I know what it takes to be successful in these interviews. Orthopaedics is one of the most difficult specialties to get into. Over the years the competition has certainly increased. Being passionate alone will not provide success in this evergrowing specialty.

Most important secret to be successful in Orthopaedic interviews, or for that matter any interview is thorough preparation.

FAIL TO PREPARE = PREPARE TO FAIL

Often interview preparation is kept for the last few days or weeks. THIS IS WRONG.

Orthopaedic interview preparation should start atleast few months before the interview.

Be thorough with every scenario in this book. Read topics mentioned in the essential reading section. Most of the scenarios mentioned in this book have been asked previously in interviews. Practice every scenario mentioned in this book again and again. You will be closer to success if you practice, practice and practice. Request Consultants or Registrars in your hospital for interview practice. Every Hospital will have Consultants who have experience of being an interviewer. And lastly, prepare for interviews as though you are preparing for an exam, seriously…

All the best. Cheers

Manjunath

ST3 orthopaedic interview process (2016)

St3 interviews in 2016 had a **longlisting process**. There was no shortlisting.
Candidates were longlisted in 2016 if they had
1. Full GMC registration by the time of starting appointment.
2. MRCS by the time of interview
3. ATLS by the time of interview
4. Achieve CT1 and CT2 competencies by the time of appointment. Candidates not in core training scheme, had to complete certificate C (Alternative Certificate of Core Competence).
5. 24 months experience in surgical specialties (not including Foundation experience), with atleast 10 months in Orthopaedics, by the time of appointment.

Interview format consisted of 5 stations.

1. Portfolio station had 2 parts:
Self assessment validation – Candidates had to submit evidence to self assessment questions before the start of the interview. Interviewers would have assessed and validated the evidence before candidates entered the station. The self assessment questions for 2016 are available on Yorkshire and Humber deanery website. [http://www.yorksandhumberdeanery.nhs.uk/media/784499/t_o_applicant_handbook_2016.pdf].

Portfolio interview (15 minutes) – 2 questions approximately, each lasting 7.5 minutes.

2. Interactive and Communication station
(15 minutes):
Candidates had to interact with actors who would roleplay a scenario. There were 2 parts to the scenario, each lasting 7.5 minutes.

3. Presentation and Handover case prioritisation (Presentation and List Planning)
(15 minutes):
Candidates were provided with a presentation topic few weeks before the interview. Candidates had to present for 3 minutes about the provided topic. This was followed by few questions about the presentation.
For the handover case or List planning (both are similar), a list of cases were provided and candidates were asked to prepare a theatre list.

4. Clinical station (15 minutes):
It consisted of 2 parts, Clinical Anatomy and Clinical knowledge, each lasting 7.5 minutes.

5. Technical skills station (15 minutes):
Candidates were asked to carry out a technical skill exercise.

Interview Stations

Portfolio station

This is split into Self Assessment validation and Portfolio interview stations.

Self assessment validation: You will need to submit portfolio containing evidence of answers to self assessment questions, before entering the station. The score generated from self assessment questions will contribute to your overall score.

TIP: Make sure the evidence for self assessment questions are identifiable easily. This will increase your chances of a higher score.

Evidence not found = Marks lost.

Remember, Interviewers have been examining candidates for that entire session and it can be taxing on them to search for information, not readily identifiable from your portfolio. Your portfolio will demonstrate organisation skills, attitude, passion for the specialty.

Time well spent in preparing portfolio will reap benefits. Remember portfolio is not 'CV'. Portfolio represents your attitude and commitment to the specialty. Discuss with your trainers and colleagues to create a portfolio which will suit yourself.

Tips for preparing portfolio:
Provide an INDEX sheet in the beginning highlighting the contents.
Use markers to bookmark your evidence/answers for the self assessment questions.
Sequence them preferably in a format to match the self assessment questions.
Headings have to be clear.
Use plastic folders or laminated sheets if possible.
Keep portfolio sleek, short and professional. Keep only relevant stuff.

Know every bit of your portfolio. You might be asked to identify some information from the portfolio, so you should be able to identify that information with ease. For example the interviewer could ask you to demonstrate DHS surgeries from portfolio.

Portfolio interview questions:
(15 minutes, 2 questions)

Tell us about yourself?
Can start with graduation and current post (keep this brief). Do not mention each and every post you have done, as it will be time consuming and will provide no extra marks. Mention your achievements or things you are proud off. It is worth matching your answers to suit the person specification. By doing this, you will present only relevant information. Remember you are selling yourself with this answer.

Mention any audits, research projects, publications, any degrees, teaching experience if you have undertaken. Mention any relevant courses and clinical experience. Mention any extracurricular work, if you have done them either within or outside NHS. Most common error is to mention your research and publications and not mention any extracurricular activities. Extracurricular activities include organising mess committee meeting, organising social events (be sensible as to which event you mention), any involvement in designing protocols, sporting achievements etc.

Your answer should demonstrate team working, reliability, commitment, management, leadership, communication skills.

The following template can be used to answer above question:

Career progression – Mention T&O experience, 2 related specialty experiences if you have them.

Courses – Mention ATLS, Fracture management etc...

Clinical experience –

Validated logbook details. Example - Number of neck of femur surgeries, distal radius fracture surgeries, ankle fracture surgeries etc done either as STS (Supervised Trainer Scrubbed) or STU (Supervised Trainer Unscrubbed). Number of validated DHS procedures in logbook has been one of the self-assessment questions in recent ST3 interviews.

Clinical management skills. Example – decision making in A&E, polytrauma management.

Academic skills – Audit, research, teaching achievements. Mention your role in each of these. You will not have enough time to discuss about individual projects for this question.

Personal skills, Probity, Commitment to specialty –

Personal skills cover various topics such as communication, decision making, teamworking, organisation skills, coping with pressure. Due to time constraints, you will not be able to provide examples for each of these qualities separately (this is in relation to question, 'tell us about yourself'?). Therefore it is best to include most of these qualities in 1 or 2 examples.

For example, with teaching experience you could demonstrate communication skills, team working, organisation skills and time management. If you have led a research project, you could also demonstrate these qualities.
Probity can be demonstrated by showing awareness of patient confidentiality, ethics in clinical practice, obtaining feedback. All of the above qualities should also fulfill criteria for commitment to specialty.

How do you suit this job? OR Why should we appoint you?

There is a degree of overlap between previous question and this one. Should know person specification for the applied job. Follow the template mentioned in previous answer to reply to this question. Mention your achievements demonstrating how you fulfil the essential criteria and some if not most of the desirable criteria in the person specification. Demonstrate with examples to show commitment, passion for the specialty, team working, management, leadership and communication skills.

Can mention any activities outside your regular schedule to demonstrate interest towards orthopaedics. These include taster sessions, plaster room sessions, relevant multidisciplinary meetings, audit and research projects, courses, attending clinics, any degrees etc.

Why do you want to do orthopaedics?
Best answered with examples. Could highlight positives in the specialty which have attracted you towards orthopaedics. For example, pain relief following hip and knee replacement or following fracture fixation might have impressed you. Or could mention some positive experience during medical school days or earlier. You could mention about some academic work such as audit or research projects, which attracted you towards the specialty.

Also mention about your personal attributes which make you well suited for this specialty. Attributes include good dexterity, hand eye coordination, anatomy interest, enjoy challenges such as making decisions in trauma, working under pressure, teamwork, teaching opportunities. Demonstrate these with examples and more importantly need to show that you thoroughly enjoy training and working in this specialty.

What do you understand by research?
Explain this in your own words, for better scores. Research is a systematic investigation to identify new knowledge OR Research is a methodological means of identifying new knowledge. There are different types of research studies. In ascending order of methodological strengths they can be classified as case series, case control studies, cohort studies, randomized control trial, systematic

review and meta analysis. Research performed in a healthcare setting is also called as clinical research.

Case series – Study of patients with similar exposure or similar outcome of interest. No control group.

Case control studies – Study compares patients with disease/outcome of interest (case) and patients without the same disease/outcome of interest (control). As the disease has already occurred, it is a retrospective study design.

Prospective cohort studies – Study compares patients who have had exposure to a particular variable with patients who have not had exposure to the same variable and follow them prospectively to identify any difference in outcome of interest/disease.

Randomised controlled trial – Study which randomly allocates patients to either an experimental group (group receiving the intervention) or control group (group not receiving the intervention or could receive placebo).

Systematic review – Methodological review of literature. It critically analyses existing literature to establish best available evidence .

Meta analysis – Statistical method of combining data from individual studies and thereby increasing the overall power, validity and reliability of the outcome.

Phases of research: for new treatments especially:
Pre clinical – Laboratory studies

Phase 1 - Testing treatment on small number of healthy volunteers

Phase 2 – Testing treatment on small number of patients

Phase 3 – Testing treatment on larger number of patients

Phase 4 – Post marketing surveillance – effectiveness of treatment continuously monitored while licensed for use in general public, to identify its safety.

What is a research proposal?
It is a summary of your proposed research. It outlines any existing knowledge, any controversies, research questions, study design, research methodology, expected duration and outcome. The proposal should also demonstrate significance of your research project.

How would you conduct a Randomised controlled trial?

Randomised controlled trial, as the name suggests, involves a methodological process of randomizing participants into study and control groups. These groups are analysed to understand the outcome of the intervention in the study group as compared to the control group.

Steps involved in setting up a RCT:
Literature search to identify existing literature about Your chosen topic.
Define Study Hypothesis.
Design study protocol, consent forms.
(If applying for research grant, send research proposal to relevant organisation)
Research Application process (Integrated Research application System)
R&D and ethical committee approvals.
Start study once R&D and Ethical approvals obtained..

Steps for applying for research funding/Grant:
Identify topic.
Design research proposal.
Identify resources and funding required.
Identify relevant funding organisation.
Submit Research proposal to the organisation.

Different types of randomisation:
Simple randomisation – Single sequence of random assignments. Example – Simple randomisation can be performed by random number tables, flipping a coin. Simple randomisation can suffer from chance bias.

Blocked randomisation – Randomise subjects into groups to create equal sample sizes. One of the variables/characteristics can be used as blocking factor. Block size has to be pre determined.

Stratified randomisation – This randomization process tries to balance the different confounding variables. Blocks/Strata are generated based on prognostic variables followed by randomization within the strata.

Strengths of RCT:
Good internal and external validity.
Robust methodology.

Drawbacks of RCT:
Time and costs.

Do you know of any RCTs published OR have you read any published RCT?
There are several good RCTs published in orthopaedic literature. Know couple of them atleast.

Examples: DRAFFT trial (Distal radius fracture fixation trial), ProFHER trial (proximal humerus fracture trial), RCTs on fracture neck of femur treatment etc……..

What is research governance?

Research Governance is a framework which sets standards in research. It also provides a means to deliver them and ensure adequate monitoring mechanisms are in place. The overall intention is to improve research and safeguard public by enhancing research performance, ethical awareness, minimizing adverse reactions and promoting good practice.
Everyone involved in research are responsible for maintaining research governance.

It consists of 5 domains:
Ethics: Primary consideration should be given to dignity, rights, safety and wellbeing of participants. Appropriate processes must be in place to obtain consent and ethical review.

Science: Thorough literature search should identify any existing evidence. Research should be original, without duplicating any other work. Data collected should be retained for an appropriate period to allow further analysis if required.

Information: Free access should be provided to information on research and its findings.

Health and Safety: Safety of all participants and research staff should be given priority and appropriate health and safety regulations must be followed.

Finance and Intellectual Property: Financial probity, respecting intellectual property rights, compliance with the rules set out by HM Treasury and ensuring adequate compensation mechanisms are in place.

(Research Governance Framework for Health and Social Care, 2005, Department of Health) – available online.

What do you understand by Clinical audit?
It is a quality improvement process that seeks to improve patient care and outcomes through systematic review of care against explicit criteria and implementation of change.

"A quality improvement process that seeks to improve patient care and outcomes through systematic review of care against explicit criteria and the implementation of change. Aspects of the structure, processes, and outcomes of care are selected and systematically evaluated against explicit criteria. Where indicated, changes are implemented at an individual, team, or service level and further monitoring is used to confirm

improvement in healthcare delivery." (Principles for Best Practice in Clinical Audit, 2002, NICE)
Remember, Interviewers are assessing your understanding of clinical audit and therefore you will need to discuss about audit in your own words rather than just mentioning the above definition, for better scores.

Essentially clinical audit involves comparing current practice with a chosen standard practice and thereby identify deficiencies in current practice to formulate an appropriate solution.

Audit cycle involves:
Identify problem/Choose topic
Choose standards (expected quality of care), set criteria (measurable outcome)
Observe current practice
Compare current practice with chosen standard
Discuss necessary changes
Implement change
Re-audit

Clinical audit is an essential part of clinical governance. It is not service evaluation or research.

Service evaluation: As the name suggests evaluates efficiency of a service through a systematic assessment of its objectives, activities, outcomes and costs. Basically it analyses if the service was a success or not. It is designed to answer the question what standard does this service achieve. Measures current service without comparison to a standard.

Difference between audit and research:

Audit	Research
Monitors existing practice to identify deficiency	Identify new knowledge
Results are locally applicable i.e., poor external validity	Results are generalizable i.e., good external validity
No randomisation	May involve randomisation
Never involves a completely new treatment	Can involve completely new treatment
Measures against standard	Tests a hypothesis

Tell us about your audit involvement Or Tell us about your research involvement.

You will need to mention about your role in each of the projects along with a brief description of each, including any background information, aims, methods, results especially any significant findings or any changes implemented.

However, if there are too many projects to discuss, you could start by mentioning that you have done 'x' number of audits and research projects and then

start discussing about the projects. By doing this, atleast you have made sure that the interviewer is aware of the number of projects you have worked hard on. You may want to start with the best ones first/most interesting ones first, as you may not have enough time to discuss all.
Use this opportunity to demonstrate your teamwork skills and leadership qualities.

What do you understand by Clinical Governance?
It is a means to maintain and continuously improve high quality of patient care in the NHS. It is a powerful tool to ensure quality of patient care is at the centre of all activities. Everyone involved in patient care is responsible for Clinical Governance, although the ultimate responsibility lies with the Chief Executive of the NHS Trust.

"A framework through which NHS organisations are accountable for continually improving the quality of their services and safeguarding high standards of care by creating an environment in which excellence in clinical care will flourish."
(Scally and Donaldson, Clinical Governance and the drive for quality improvement in the new NHS in England, BMJ, 1998)

Remember, Interviewers are assessing your understanding of clinical Governance and therefore you will need to discuss about Clinical Governance in your own words rather than just mentioning the above definition, for better scores.

Its main components include:
Education and Training - It is vital for all healthcare staff to undergo regular training and Continuous Profession Development, as knowledge gained previously can be outdated.

Clinical audit – Ensure a regular audit system is in place to maintain quality of care. To learn lessons and formulate appropriate changes.

Evidence Based care and effectiveness – Evidence Based Practice is essential to provide the best possible care to patients, based on the best available evidence. Effectiveness measure the extent to which a particular intervention works.

Research and development – Research is essential to identify new treatments which can improve the quality of care provided. Systems have to be in place to ensure critical appraisal of literature, project management, development of protocols, and implementation of strategies can take place.

Risk management – Minimise risk to Patients, Healthcare staff and Organisation. To ensure systems are regularly reviewed. To learn from adverse events and appropriate actions are taken to prevent recurrence.

Patient confidentiality – To ensure patient information is maintained securely and only available to relevant staff. To ensure patient data is not misused.

Openness – There has to be a culture of openness and honesty among Healthcare staff with patients, colleagues, employers and organisations. Systems have to be in place to support and encourage such behavior.

Remember everyone is responsible for clinical governance.
Give example of your involvement in clinical governance such as involvement in any clinical audit or research projects, teaching, evidence based care, maintaining patient confidentiality, risk management etc…

What is evidence based medicine?
"Evidence based medicine is the process of systematically finding, appraising, and using contemporaneous research findings as the basis for clinical decisions."
(Rosenberg W, Donald A. Evidence based medicine: an approach to clinical problem-solving. BMJ 1995; 310: 1122–1126)
Essentially it involves making clinical decisions based on best available evidence.

Evidence based medicine process (Rosenberg W, Donald A. BMJ 1995)

- Formulate an answerable clinical question
- Literature search for evidence
- Critical appraisal of the evidence
- Act on the evidence

Formulate an answerable question:
'PICO' format often used.
P – Patient/Problem – Patient or problem being addressed.
I – Intervention – Intervention being considered
C – Comparison – Is the intervention being compared with another comparative intervention (not always required)
O – Outcome – what is the outcome of interest

Literature search:
Using keywords relevant to the question, literature databases (example – pubmed, Cochrane, Embase etc) are searched. Unpublished literature will also need to be searched to improve reliability and validity of the outcome.

Critical appraisal:
Once literature is identified, it will need to be critically appraised to assess how reliable and valid the outcome is. Several appraisal tools are also available.

Act on the evidence:
Based on the outcome and its appraisal findings, healthcare professionals can decide whether evidence needs to be implemented or not.

Advantages of evidence based medicine:
Knowledge gained about the problem.
Gained experience in literature search and analysing literature.
Improves confidence in decision making.
Effective use of resources.
Better understanding about the rationale behind clinical decisions.
Combination of above leads to improved patient care.

Need to know examples of evidence based decision making, to improve your score. Examples include NICE guidance for fracture neck of femur treatment, NICE guidelines for thromboprophylaxis post hip and knee replacements etc...

Levels of evidence: (Oxford, UK, CEBM Levels of Evidence, 2011)

Level 1 – Well designed RCT or systematic review of RCT.
Level 2 – Prospective cohort study or Systematic review of cohort studies or low quality RCT(without adequate randomization, <80% follow up).
Level 3 – Case control studies or systematic review of case control studies.

Level 4 – Case series
Level 5 – Expert opinion

Tell us about your experience of teamwork? OR What do you know about teamwork?
Teamwork is a process of collaborative working to achieve a common goal. Healthcare staff are interdependent on each other to provide the best possible patient care. Teamwork is witnessed in every aspect of day to day care such as ward work, clinics, operating theatres, on calls, teaching, audit and research projects. Networking and collaboration have become essential parts of modern NHS. Examples include trauma regional networks, research networks.

Requirements for successful teamwork:
Have clear objectives.
Should know each other's role and responsibility.
Identify and prevent barriers to collaborative working.
Active and constructive communication between team members.
Learn from reflection.
Mutual respect.

Advantages of teamwork:
Shared decision making.
Shared ideas.
Shared responsibility.
Increase mutual understanding.

Reduce Individual workload.
Increase overall efficiency.

Example:
Having been part of the trauma team at a Major Trauma Centre, I have attended few trauma calls in A&E. This experience made me realise the importance of teamwork. All members of the trauma team had clear objectives and knew each other's responsibility. There was active communication between members. Team members were flexible in their roles and supported each other quite well. Being a trauma team member has also helped me understand the importance of collaborative working, as witnessed with the Trauma regional networks. This has certainly improved the overall care of major trauma patients.

How do you see yourself in 10 years?
Due to my immense interest in both academic and clinical orthopaedics, I would have participated in several research projects, presentations, publications and clinical duties over the next 10 years. At 10 years, I would be a Consultant in subspecialty of my choice and would be leading research and audit projects. Will ensure patients are at the centre of my decision making, which will be based on principles of evidence based medicine. Will optimise theatre and clinic space to ensure junior staff have adequate training opportunities. Due to my interest in teaching and training, I would

have taken up the role of educational supervisor along with organising teaching programmes for medical students and junior staff. Would consider becoming an ATLS instructor.

I would have completed courses on management and leadership. I will be involved in making management decisions as personally I feel Clinicians are good managers. Will take part in service development projects such as setting protocols and patient information leaflets. My practice will utilise available resources efficiently to maximize cost effectiveness. At 10 years, as a Consultant I would have crossed the initial settling in period and therefore will be in an advantageous position to guide other members of my team.

Tell us about your teaching experience?

Teaching is an essential part of Medical practice. Good teaching is not just about teaching, it is about motivating students to learn as well as showing them how to learn. One needs to be passionate about teaching to enjoy the overall experience.

As suggested by GMC Good Medical Practice 2013:
'Teaching, training, appraising and assessing doctors and students are important for the care of patients now and in the future. If you are involved in

teaching you must develop the skills, attitudes and practices of a competent teacher.'

Skills of a competent teacher:

1. Be a good listener – being patient and listening is essential for effective communication.

2. Be a good communicator – Should express thoughts clearly and be informative. Obtain regular feedback to improve the overall process.

3. Being flexible – Having a strict agenda, may not be beneficial always, as the teaching needs to be tapered to the students requirements.

4. Use teaching aids - "What I hear, I forget; what I see, I remember; what I do, I know".
Pictures, practical demonstrations can be more effective in certain situations.

5. Understand students requirements – Most important.

6. Exhibit professionalism – Being organized, maintaining time and schedule.

7. Being inspirational.

Of course, teaching is also a learning experience. Several transferable skills can be acquired from teaching including communication skills, organization skills and time management skills. Not to mention the additional knowledge gained from the teaching experience. In healthcare setting, it is vital to ensure patient care is not compromised by teaching schedule (Good Medical Practice, GMC, 2013).

Teaching methods can be broadly split into
Teacher centered methods – lectures, direct instructions.
Student centered methods – problem based learning, group projects.

Example answer:
Throughout my training, I have been actively involved in teaching. In the last year I have organized and managed departmental teaching. I was involved in teaching medical students in clinics and wards. My teaching topics have included fracture neck of femur, ankle fractures, osteoarthritis. Have utilised different teaching methods including didactic style teaching, problem based approach and group projects. Teaching method is generally tapered to suit the student population I am teaching. My teaching tends to be interactive, as I prefer active involvement of my audience. Personally I have always gained from my teaching experience. It has improved my communications skills and knowledge. Through a process of regular feedback and assessments, my overall teaching experience has improved. As evidence of my teaching, I have attached feedback and assessments forms from my teaching session.

I have also obtained a post graduate degree in teaching.

How will you organise teaching in your department?

This question analyses organisation skills and team working in addition to teaching skills.

Example answer – I will discuss with my colleagues, trainers and students to plan the teaching syllabus and also to identify a suitable time for teaching medical students. I will ensure patient care is not compromised during teaching hours. I will discuss with the postgraduate department to arrange a suitable place and time for teaching. Will ensure teaching syllabus covers relevant topics of interest. Teaching schedule with relevant study material will be provided atleast few weeks in advance so that students have sufficient time to prepare. Will discuss with my colleagues to ensure there are no individual concerns with the teaching programme.

Learning objectives will be outlined at the beginning of every session to make the purpose and content explicit. Students will be encouraged to interact actively in these sessions. Also, the syllabus will cover a wide spectrum of knowledge, as students can vary in their understanding about the subject. Presentations will be mainly powerpoint based. Group discussions will be encouraged to promote active thinking. Handouts will be provided at the

end of the session regarding the next teaching. Students will also be requested to fill out anonymized feedback forms after every teaching session, to improve the overall experience. Future teaching will be restructured if necessary based upon student feedback.
I will then reflect on the teaching session, make an appropriate action plan and maintain a record in portfolio.

***Are doctors good managers? Tell us about your management experience*?**

There has been a shortage of doctors in management roles in United Kingdom. Experience from United States has shown that most of the top performing hospitals in the States, have doctors leading the management role. Sir Francis report about failings of Mid Staffordshire NHS Trust highlighted poor relations between managers and clinicians.

There is raising focus to engage doctors in managerial roles. Doctors tend to prioritise patient care over other issues. Whereas managers focus more on maximising resources within available budget. Managers have no direct contact with patients and therefore their decisions tend to be based on charts and various analyses. I therefore think Doctors are good if not better managers, as doctors tend to include patient care in the decision making process. Doctors are in a position to act both as managers interested to minimise losses and also as clinicians interested in patient care. This balance is essential if we have to place patients at the centre of our decision making. Over the years, more and more clinicians are involved in managerial roles.

Some of the barriers for doctors to take up managerial roles include insufficient exposure to management roles during training years, fear of losing clinical skills, insufficient time to balance clinical and managerial duties.

Yes I have also been involved in managing a research project. Along with designing and organizing the research study, I was involved in managing the funding for the research project, recruiting the research team and participants, allocating duties, setting timelines and regular discussion with team members to check on progress. I had to ensure that the project was completed within the available resources. I enjoyed this challenge thoroughly and certainly has added to my personal attributes such as team working, communication skills and management skills.

What is the future of orthopaedics?

The future of Orthopaedics is bright as the current generation of orthopaedic surgeons are thriving hard to maintain the highest standards of patient care. In future, more and more surgeons will consider managerial responsibilities. The demand for Orthopaedic surgeons is certainly on the rise, with ageing population and increasing patient demands. This will inturn increase financial costs and burden. Therefore cost effectiveness will play a pivotal role in decision making. Orthopaedic Surgeons seem to be preparing for these challenges as evidenced by the various ongoing research projects to improve quality of patient care as well as overall efficiency. Audit tools are in place to monitor practices. The rapid improvement in technology has increased the accuracy of targeted treatment, for example use of navigation in joint replacements.

More and more procedures are being done as outpatient procedures or short stay procedures to minimize costs. As mentioned in Professor Briggs report, “Get it Right first time” (GIRFT, 2012) services could be centralized to pool Surgeons and improve surgical exposure for selected operations (example – revision surgeries). This will also decrease implant costs, as with larger numbers being used at a single centre, prices could be negotiated better. There will be increasing scrutiny to ensure better patient care. Over the years training and assessments have become increasingly robust and this will continue to become more robust. This will also increase the amount of supervised training. Collaborations and networking will increase in future to provide patients with the best possible care.

Tell us about your strengths and weaknesses?
Best answered with some examples. Even better if you have any evidence in your portfolio to substantiate this. Evidence includes certificates, feedback forms, assessments. Can mention any of your strengths. If you have a number of strengths, you could mention those briefly but then focus onto your main strength. Need to justify why you think this is your main strength. No particular strength scores better than others.

For weakness, your ability to identify areas for improvement and implement appropriate actions will be assessed. You will need to show what lessons you have learnt and how this has changed your practice. Telling your weakness will not deduct points, as long as you demonstrate what steps you have taken to overcome this. Again as with strengths, if you have any evidence to substantiate your answers, you could score better.
For weakness, you could use "POOR" type proforma to answer.
[POOR – problem, obstacles, opportunities, remedy]

How do you deal with negative feedback and criticism?
Interviewers are assessing your ability to learn from feedback and cope with stress. "POOR" [POOR – problem, obstacles, opportunities, remedy] proforma can be used.

You need to demonstrate a commitment towards learning, positive attitude and enthusiasm. Provide examples from your experience. I am sure everyone would have received negative feedback at some point. Mention the negative feedback and reason you received this. Then go on to show steps you have taken to overcome this weakness with the available opportunities. Demonstrate how this has changed your practice or attitude or personal skills.

Example answer: I take negative feedback positively. Being a self motivated person, negative feedback makes me to strive harder and more efficiently. For example, during my initial years of training, I was not presenting well at meetings as I tended to be a bit shy during presentations. This was identified by one of my Consultants, who provided a negative feedback about my presentation. This motivated me to work harder to improve my presentation skills. Subsequently, I attended a presentation course, performed more presentations and obtained regular feedback from various sources after every presentation. I also started focusing on my body language and eye contact, during my presentation. With regular practice and feedback, my presentation skills eventually improved. This has also improved my confidence enormously.

What is the most successful thing you have done?

Discuss about a single event, of your choice. It could be an academic achievement, clinical achievement or managerial achievement. Could be an achievement outside orthopaedics. You will need to discuss as to why this achievement was important, what was your involvement, what were the implications, any lessons learnt.
This is also an opportunity to demonstrate your personal traits such as leadership qualities, teamwork, management experience, communication skills, enthusiasm, positive attitude etc.

Is communication skill important OR What do you know about effective communication?

Good Communication is essential part of Modern NHS. In current climate of austerity, good communication will improve efficiency and cost effectiveness. It will provide a more satisfying interaction with colleagues and better time management. It will most certainly improve quality of patient care.

Communication skill needs to be practiced. Make use of every opportunity to improve on communication. It is vital to know your limitations and ways to improve them. Certainly good communication provides a major advantage in day to day practice, presentations and interviews. Poor

Communication is the most common reason for litigation and complaints in NHS.
GMC (Good Medical Practice 2013) has suggested for communication to be effective "You must give patients the information they want or need to know in a way they can understand".

For communication to be effective, it has to be clear and focused. It has to be tapered to the other person's requirements as it will keep them more engaged. Positive body language is important for effective communication, maintaining eye contact shows your interest in the discussion (applies to interviews as well). For communication to be effective, you have to be a good listener. Listen and empathise with patients.

Steps for effective communication skills:

1. Obtain information by using open ended questions.
2. Listen and Understand patient beliefs and concerns.
3. Provide relevant information in patient's language.
4. Arrive at a shared decision.
5. Summarise and conclude.

You can also demonstrate your communication skills by providing example about a situation where your communication made a difference to the final outcome. For example, helping patients make an informed decision, by communicating about the treatment effectively.

Have you had any leadership roles? Or What do you know about leadership?

It has been widely recognized that better leadership leads to better care. All doctors have to perform Leadership role at some stage.

There are 2 types of leadership. Formal leadership and shared leadership (GMC, Good Medical Practice,2012).

Formal leaders are accountable for the performance of their organization or team.

Shared leadership occurs when the responsibility is shared by all team members.

Qualities of a good leader:

Ability to motivate others.

Ability to delegate

Assertiveness

Empathy

Effective communicator.

Difference between Leadership and Management:

Though managers and leaders can have overlapping roles, there are certain differences between the two. A leader is able to innovate, inspire and make changes.

Whereas managers focus mainly on the processes and systems in place and try to maintain them.

While leaders rely on peoples trust, managers rely on controlling them.

Examples of leadership roles include, leading a research or audit project, leading trauma calls, leading MDT etc...It is important to explain your role and experience gained, including challenges faced and lessons learnt. A good leader learns from feedback.

What do you understand by Professional integrity at work?

Professional integrity is acting within the social and moral values of the profession. To follow the code of ethics relevant to the profession. In the wider sense, it means treating others the way you want to be treated. To maintain professional integrity, it is essential to familiarize with rules and regulations that govern the profession (GMC Good Medical Practice, 2013).

Its elements include probity, confidentiality, personal credibility. Professional integrity encompasses working in good partnership with patients and respecting their rights, maintaining confidentiality of sensitive information, following rules and regulations in a consistent non biased manner, maintaining ethics. Revalidation process ensures that work is performed within set guidelines.

***What do you know about Revalidation**?*
(www.gmc-uk.org)
Revalidation is a process of ensuring that all licensed doctors are up to date and fit to practice in their chosen field and able to provide a good quality of care. Revalidation is performed once every five years. To ensure licensed doctors are up to date and fit to practice, regular appraisal systems are in place. A designated Responsible Officer will assess your portfolio and send recommendation to GMC. The following types of supporting information is required by the GMC:
Continuing professional development
Quality improvement activity
Significant events
Feedback from colleagues
Feedback from patients
Review of complaints and compliments

Revalidation was confirmed by the Secretary of State for Health on 3rd December 2012. The first revalidation cycle was planned in stages. Majority of responsible officers and other medical leaders were revalidated by March 2013. About a fifth of licensed doctors were revalidated between April 2013 and the end of March 2014. The remaining licensed doctors by the end of March 2018.

Advantages of revalidation:
Doctors are better regulated.
Ensures Doctors keep up to date, as it is a ongoing process.

Patient feedback forms are part of the appraisal and revalidation. Thereby it provides extra confidence to patients, that their Doctors are regularly checked.

What do you understand by Appraisal and assessments?

Assessment is evaluation of knowledge or skills against objective standards. Assessment is primarily performed for the service provider/Supervisor to monitor competence of the assesse. It can be judgmental.

Whereas appraisal is a structured dialogue between a appraisee and appraiser. Appraisal provides feedback, charts ongoing progress and identifies a developmental plan primarily aimed at improvement of the appraisee. It is non-judgmental. It forms one of the elements of Clinical Governance. It is linked closely with revalidation.

NHS appraisal has been in place since 2002, following the Bristol and Shipman inquiries, to include performance review in appraisals. GMC in its Good Medical Practice framework suggested four core domains of Appraisal, which also form the basis for revalidation.

1. Knowledge, skills and performance
1a. Maintain your professional performance.
1b. Apply knowledge and experience to practice.

1c. Ensure that all documentation formally recording your work is clear, accurate and legible.
2. Safety and Quality
2a. Contribute to and comply with systems to protect patients.
2b. Respond to risks to safety.
2c. Protect patients and colleagues from any risk posed by your health.

3. Communication, Partnership and Teamwork
3a. Communicate effectively.
3b. Work constructively with colleagues and delegate effectively.
3c. Establish and maintain partnerships with patients.

4. Maintaining Trust
4a. Show respect for patients.
4b. Treat patients and colleagues fairly and without discrimination.
4c. Act with honesty and integrity.

How will you reduce NHS costs? OR How will you reduce NHS expenses?

When asked to solve issues, have a structured reply. A structured reply makes your response professional and knowledgeable. One of the ways of structuring is by creating a "POOR" format.

POOR proforma:

P – Problem – What are you trying to solve

O – Obstacles – What are the obstacles hindering progress or responsible for creating the Problem "P"

O – Opportunities – what are the available opportunities to solve the problem

R – Remedy – Finally, what is the solution for the problem "P"

Creating "POOR" format for the above question:

P – (Problem) How to reduce NHS costs

O- (Obstacles)
Delayed discharge
Readmission rates
Deficient human resource
Surgical implant costs
Patient complications
Etc……..

O- (Opportunities)
Identify opportunities locally by performing audits, discussion with frontline staff, colleagues and stakeholders.

R – (Remedy)

Identify patients for discharge early, timely discharge summaries.
Reduce readmission rates by performing audits to identify the reason for readmission and implement changes.
Insufficient human resource can lead to relying on bank/locum staff.
Decrease variation in the type of implants used to get a better deal with the implant companies (GIRFT report, Prof. Tim Briggs, 2015)
Minimise complications (GIRFT report, Prof. Tim Briggs, 2015)
Minimise losses, improve efficiency.
Perform regular audits to monitor performance.
Perform research to identify new knowledge and improve efficiency.

(Important reading - GIRFT report, Prof. Tim Briggs 2015, available online at http://www.gettingitrightfirsttime.com/)

Using a structured format makes problem solving easy. You do not need to answer all the points mentioned in the above example. You will be fine as long as you can articulate the structure and mention some of the points.

What do you know about payment by results?
(www.gov.uk)
Payment by results (PbR) is a payment system in NHS England whereby Commissioners pay healthcare providers for each patient episode taking into account the complexity of the patient's healthcare needs. The two fundamental features of PbR are nationally determined currencies and tariffs. PbR currently covers the majority of acute healthcare in hospitals, with national tariffs for admitted patient care, outpatient attendances, accident and emergency and some outpatient procedures. For example, £5,323 for a hip operation.

Block contracts were in place before PbR, wherein a fixed amount of money was paid to hospitals irrespective of the number of patients treated or their complexity.

Advantages of PbR:
1. The money follows the patient.
2. If Hospitals can provide standard care at lower costs than the National price, the profits made can be retained by the Hospital.
3. Pay Hospitals for the amount of work done. So Hard working hospitals can get paid more. This can also reduce waiting times.
4. It focusses towards providing better quality of care and innovation

5. To discourage poor performance, commissioners and NHS providers have a list of 'never events' for which no payment will be made.

What is best practice tariff?
(www.gov.uk)
For certain procedures which have strong evidence defining good practice, 'best practice tariffs' have been introduced to improve quality by reducing unexplained variation and universalising best practice, in England. The purpose being to incentivize and adequately reimburse providers for the costs of high quality care. The idea is to maintain and improve high quality of care for these procedures. The current list of best practice tariff procedures include cholecystectomy, cataract, fragility hip fracture care, acute stroke care, interventional radiology, primary total hip and knee replacements, adult renal dialysis, Transient Ischaemic Attacks (TIAs), paediatric medicine and day cases in breast surgery, general surgery, gynaecology, orthopaedics and urology.

Best practice tariff for fracture neck of femur:
Patients admitted with fracture neck of femur in England have to fulfill certain criteria to be eligible for best practice tariff, wherein a £1,335 uplift is awarded per patient.
Criteria include: admission using an agreed assessment protocol, Surgery within 36 hours of admission, shared care between orthopaedics and

geriatrics, assessment by senior geriatrician within 72 hours, documentation of both pre- and post-operative abbreviated mental test (AMT) scores, geriatrician-led multi-disciplinary rehabilitation, a falls assessment, and a bone health assessment. Studies have consistently shown these criteria to have a positive influence on the outcome.

What do you know about Francis Enquiry report?

The Francis enquiry report examined causes of failure at Mid Staffordshire NHS Foundation Trust between 2005 – 2009. The report made 290 recommendations. The second report was published in 2013 (first report 2010). The report essentially stressed on openness, transparency, honesty, probity, improving support for compassionate and committed caring and stronger healthcare leadership.

In 2015, a report titled "Culture Change in the NHS" was published to showcase the steps taken by the Government following Francis Report into Mid Staffordshire failings.

In brief, a new and rigorous inspection regime was introduced for hospitals, GPs and adult social care. Three Chief Inspectors were since appointed. More staff were hired at Special measures Trusts with changes in board-level leadership. The report also emphasised the need to maintain vigilance and continue improvements.

What are 'Special measures' NHS Trusts?
If there are concerns regarding quality of patient care provided by any NHS trusts, they are put into 'special measures'. This is done to offer those Trusts support to improve and also to provide the public the ability to hold them to account.
Some of the Special measures include:
The 'special measure' trust will be partnered with a high-performing NHS foundation trust or NHS trust to help deliver improvements.
Regularly updated action plan will be published on the NHS Choices website, detailing the progress being made.
The trust will have an improvement director – appointed by and accountable to NHS Improvement.
Foundation trusts can lose their autonomy.
The leadership of the trust will be reviewed as appropriate.
(www.nhs.uk)

Difference between NHS Foundation Trusts and NHS Trusts
(www.nhs.uk, www.england.nhs.uk)

	NHS foundation trust	NHS trust
Government involvement	Not directed by government, therefore more freedom to make strategic decisions	Directed by government
Regulation: Financial Quality	 Monitor CQC*	 Trust Development Authority CQC*
Finance	Free to make their own financial decisions according to an agreed framework set out in law and by regulators. Can retain and reinvest surpluses	Financially accountable to government

*CQC (Care Quality Commission): Independent regulator for health and social care in England. It monitors the quality of care provided by hospitals, care homes, dental and GP surgeries. It also publishes its findings and ratings to help public make the right choice.

Essential reading:

1. Briggs report – "Getting it right first time"
(http://www.gettingitrightfirsttime.com/downloads/briggsreporta4_fin.pdf)

2. Professor Donald Berwick report – 'A Promise to learn – a commitment to act; Improving the safety of patients in England"
(https://www.gov.uk/government/uploads/system/uploads/attachment_data/file/226703/Berwick_Report.pdf)

3. Department of Health "Better Procurement, Better Value, Better Care"
(https://www.gov.uk/government/uploads/system/uploads/attachment_data/file/226835/procurement_development_programme_for_NHS.pdf)

4. 7 day NHS
https://www.england.nhs.uk/ourwork/qual-clin-lead/7-day-week/

5. National Joint Registry
www.njrcentre.org.uk

6. Structure of NHS

(www.nhs.uk)

These essential papers should cover most of the portfolio questions regarding management and cost effectiveness. Read and Quote them appropriately when answering questions, as it will improve your scores.

Interactive and Comunication stations

Introduction

Remember the following mnemonic "**UR TABLE PC**" for all interactive and communication stations. Practice stations using this mnemonic, you will find these stations easier to score marks.

U - Understand the question/scenario
R - Roleplay (get into the situation, yes seriously!!)

T – Task (What is your task. This station is about your talking skills)
A - Ask questions (Seek more information)
B - Body language (Maintain eye contact, be professional)
L - Listen (Very important, pay attention and listen patiently)
E - Empathise (Understand the feelings, concerns of the actor)

P – Plan (Have a plan for the future at the end of the conversation. Do not end your conversation abruptly)
C - Clarity (Be clear with your discussion, ask the actor if everything was clear and if they need any

more clarification/information. Could do this at any time during conversation, but definitely at the end)

When practicing with colleagues, ask colleagues to score/critique against each of the criteria described in UR TABLE PC. This will certainly improve your overall score in communication stations.

Scenario 1A: It is your first day as ST3. F2 wants to discuss about a patient with back pain and urinary symptoms. It is 5PM and you are on call. You are working in a DGH without any spine service.

This station will assess your history taking skills, listening ability, communication with junior colleagues, body language and thought process. (Remember communication stations are not just about communication). You will need to be polite when you communicate with colleagues, understand the situation and be able to make a sensible decision under pressure.

Apply principles of "UR TABLE PC" to this scenario,
U (Understand the scenario) – Understand the question, it is about back pain with urinary symptoms (cauda equine syndrome)
R (Roleplay) – Get into on call registrar mode. Ensure privacy and chaperone present (could mention this in most stations).

T (Task) – Discuss with F2, obtain as much information as possible.
A (Ask)– Ask history and examination findings, ask if F2 has any concerns.
B (Body language) – confident and polite, maintain eye contact. (This statement will be repeated in every scenario. It is amazing how often doctors forget to maintain eye contact when discussing with patients or actors).
L (Listen) – Listen carefully (looks bad if you ask something which F2 has already informed)
E (Empathise) – Understand concerns of F2
(Accept you are also concerned about the patient. Appreciate the F2 for performing a good assessment. It is important to provide positive feedback, as it will enhance the F2 doctor's training experience.)

P (Plan) – Make a plan at the end of this conversation
(Plan would be for you to go and assess the patient, as you are concerned about possible Cauda Equina Syndrome and subsequently to formulate a management plan which would involve arranging MRI scan/discussion with spinal surgeons).
C (Clarity) – Be clear with your plan and discussion. Ask F2 if they have any questions.

Scenario 1B – For the above patient, You suspect cauda equine syndrome. However there is no out of hours MRI scan facility at your Hospital. Also the local spine service is about 40 miles. You are on the phone to Orthopaedic consultant on call.

Again apply principles of UR TABLE PC.
U – Understand the change in scenario
R – You are still the on call registrar

T – Have all the relevant facts to discuss with your Consultant beforehand. Make a mental plan using *SBAR handover protocol, used widely in most hospitals. Start communication with your consultant.
A – Not much of asking here from your side, as consultant will be interested to know about actions you have taken. At the end of your conversation you will need to ask if there is anything else to be done.
B – Be confident with your conversation
L – Listen carefully, if asked any questions answer accordingly.
E – Make your concerns about cauda equine syndrome obvious to the on call Consultant.

P – You will mention this as part of the SBAR protocol. However, if you forget, the on-call Consultant will ask for your plan to assess decision making skills. You can mention something along the lines that you think patient needs urgent MRI scan, to rule out Cauda Equina Syndrome. Mention about lack of MRI facility at local Hospital. Could mention that you have already discussed with nearby spine centre regarding this patient and suggest their plan, as happens in real life. You could also mention that you have discussed with the nearest Hospital with available MRI facility to see if they could perform the scan. (Read about Cauda Equina syndrome in the clinical section)

When asked to discuss with Consultant over phone, they will be interested to know your actions and management plan. Have a structure and sequence when informing about patients. This will increase your score. If your plan is wrong, Consultant will suggest otherwise. A wrong plan will not fail you in this station, don't worry. You are being assessed for the way you interact, which should be logical and methodical.

***SBAR protocol:** Useful when handing over patients to colleagues or informing about patients to Seniors/Colleagues, as in this station.
S – Situation
Introduce yourself, check you are speaking to the correct person, inform patient details.
B – Background
Reason for patient's attendance to Hospital, any past medical history, any bowel/bladder symptoms.
A – Assessment
Your assessment of patient. Examination findings. In this scenario, mention lumbar spine examination

findings, per rectal examination findings. (In trauma scenarios, start with ATLS type description – ABCDE). Mention Differential diagnosis depending upon scenario. Any relevant Investigations required. Also mention any relevant patient concerns.
R – Remedy
Your management plan. MRI. As MRI not available at your hospital discussion with nearby MRI unit/ discussion with spinal surgeons.

Scenario 2A. Patient Mr.Smith who is 85 years old, with severe dementia had Right DHS performed by yourself 2 days back. You are currently ST3 registrar. Mr.Smith has now developed chest infection. Daughter (next of kin) is angry and feels quality of care provided to Mr.Smith was inadequate. You are the doctor looking after the patient and have made arrangements to discuss patient care with daughter.

Apply principles of "UR TABLE PC" to this scenario. Actors can be aggressive sometimes in these types of stations. But you will need to remain calm!! and concentrate on the task. This station will assess your ability to deal with complex and sensitive situation. It will also assess your ability to communicate under stress.

UR TABLE PC

U – Understand the question, it is about dealing with angry relative.
R – Get into the role.

T – Introduce yourself and confirm daughter's details. Discuss with daughter. Do not give false information.
A – Ask about daughter's knowledge regarding ongoing treatment and then you could start discussing the current episode of chest infection and treatment. Also ask if daughter has any concerns or anything in particular she is worried about.
B – Body language – be confident and polite, maintain eye contact.
L – Listen and reply carefully (Daughter can ask questions such as why did a junior doctor perform surgery on dad? Is chest infection related to surgery? Will dad recover? ....be prepared)
E – Understand concerns of daughter. Be sensitive and empathetic. (Can add statements such as, we are also concerned about Mr.Smith's chest infection and we are doing our best. Hence we have discussed with our medical colleagues who have kindly reviewed Mr.Smith and have suggested antibiotic and oxygen therapy. They have suggested that he should be able to make a good recovery) Do not address Mr.Smith as 'patient' in front of daughter.

P – Make a future plan for management at the end of this conversation. Provide reassurance. Be optimistic.
C – Be clear with your plan and ask if everything was clear. Ask if she has any more concerns. Provide ward contact details at end of conversation, so that she could contact you through the ward, if she has any more concerns.

Scenario 2B – Mr.Smith is now 2 weeks following Right DHS fixation. He was complaining of increasing right hip pain. Therefore, he underwent xrays which suggested that the DHS has cut through the femoral head and your Consultant is planning for removal of DHS and conversion to THR. Intraoperative Hip Xray suggested that the DHS lag screw was superior and anterior in the femoral neck. Daughter has arrived to the hospital at your request and is unaware of DHS failure. You will need to discuss with the patient regarding your Consultant's decision. (XRAYS are usually kept on the table, so look around)

This station will test sensitive issues such as probity, honesty, breaking bad news. Maintaining patient's trust, acting with integrity and honesty are essential duties of a doctor recommended by the GMC (Good Medical practice, 2013). Medical profession is in a tough phase at present. Patient dissatisfaction and litigation has been on the rise for the last few years. Most of this is secondary to poor communication and not being honest with patients. This station is approached using structure 'UR TABLE PC'.

U – Understand the question, it is about breaking bad news and discussing failed surgery.

R – Get into the role

T – Discuss with relative. Do not give false information. Start by obtaining information regarding awareness of daughter about ongoing treatment. Then mention that you have some bad news (warning shot - I am afraid, I have some bad news for you). Pause...Allow daughter time to understand that the news is not good. Then continue with discussing about current situation and failed treatment. Better to explain failed surgery with xrays, if available.

A – Ask daughter if the information was clear. Also ask if she is alright and if she needs anyone else with her during this discussion (This applies to any breaking bad news scenario).

B – Body language – be confident and polite. Maintain eye contact.

L – Listen and communicate carefully (Daughter can ask questions such as why did a junior doctor perform surgery on dad? Is failure because junior doctor operated, why was Consultant absent? Is THR major surgery? Will dad recover? Daughter might say she is not happy discussing with junior doctor as her Dad had poor outcome from a junior doctor ....be prepared)

Example answer for- Why did a junior doctor operate on my Dad? Why did surgery fail?
Answer – I can understand as to why you are asking this question. I would have asked a similar question if I were in your place. Let me please explain this. I agree that surgery was performed by a junior doctor. However, junior doctor does not imply an incompetent doctor. All doctors are assessed for their competencies by Consultants. It is only when the Consultant feels confident about the junior doctors ability to operate, they will be allowed to operate independently. A similar situation happened with Mr.Smith and a junior doctor was allowed to operate. Do you have any questions at this stage.

With fracture neck of femur, unfortunately not all surgeries are successful. Failure happens usually due to a combination of factors. With Mr.Smith, I agree that the surgical fixation was suboptimal. Whether this alone led to failure of fixation or where there were other contributory factors such as osteoporosis, age, failure of blood supply to femoral head at the time of fracture, is difficult to say.
So the current situation is that the fixation has moved and therefore has led to failure. This will need surgery to remove the implant and perform a total hip replacement. We have had a discussion regarding Mr.Smith in the department and the best treatment was considered to be a hip replacement.

Yes this is a bigger operation that the first one as it involves removing the implant and providing an artificial hip joint. But it has to be done to provide pain relief and also to help Mr.Smith to mobilise. Was this discussion helpful and clear? Do you have any further questions? If you remember any further questions later, please let the ward staff know, so that we can have a discussion again.

If daughter suggests that she is not happy or satisfied with your explanation, you should offer arranging a discussion with the Consultant.

E – Empathise – Daughter is rightly worried at this stage as her Dad had failed surgery. Also she might be under the impression that failure occurred because a junior doctor operated on her dad. Understand concerns of daughter. Be sensitive and empathetic. (Can add statements such as, yes we are also concerned about Mr.Smith and we are doing our best).

P – Make a future plan. In this case THR. Mention it is common procedure though it is considered as a major procedure. (Know complications of THR, as daughter might ask)

C – Be clear with your plan and discussion. Ask the patient if she has any more concerns.

Scenario 3. Patient Mr.John, 95 year old with severe dementia, had hemiarthroplasty 1 week back. But has gradually deteriorated. Has significant co morbidities. Medical team have decided that patient is not a suitable candidate for CPR. You have been asked to discuss regarding resuscitation status with son (next of kin).
The same question can be to discuss resuscitation with the patient himself.

This is again a sensitive topic, which needs a lot of practice.

This station will assess your communication skills, ability to discuss sensitive information, empathy and clinical knowledge regarding DNA CPR. Be genuine with your answers. Good clinical practice includes shared decision making between patients and clinicians. Talk along lines such as resuscitation status is a type of advance directive. DNACPR is not about abandonment but to allow a dignified and peaceful natural death Explain current treatment and also explain that multidisciplinary teams are involved including physicians. We feel that resuscitation will not provide a good quality of life however can prolong life. Explain CPR can be a traumatic process to patient. Can sustain rib fractures and can be painful. The ultimate decision is with the patient/next of kin. Your role is to discuss why you and your team feel DNAR is appropriate for this gentleman. You can also provide some time suggesting that they do not need to decide right now. You can also provide some leaflets from the hospital explaining about DNAR. Also provide your contact details at the end, if they need any more clarification.

Structure 'UR TABLE PC' can be used.
U – Understand the question, it is about discussing with son about resuscitation status/DNACPR (Do Not Attempt Cardio Pulmonary Resuscitation).
R – Get into the role, ensure privacy and chaperone present.

T – Introduce yourself, confirm son's details. Start discussion. It is good to start with understanding son's knowledge regarding Mr.John's current status.
A – Ask about son's awareness of Mr.John's deterioration. Ask about son's expectations.
B – Confident, polite, maintain eye contact (you should all know this by now)
L – Listen to son's expectations/concerns.
E – Empathise, explain facts about DNACPR.

P – Mention DNACPR. Patients and relatives feel that DNACPR means stopping treatment. Mention that active treatment will still continue until the patient stops breathing or heart stops working.
C – Be clear

DNACPR guidelines UK:

Patient with mental capacity to make decision have the right to accept or refuse DNACPR. Such decisions have to be respected. Discussion in advance is an important part of good clinical care. There is no need to discuss about DNACPR if the patient is unlikely to sustain a cardio pulmonary arrest.

In a patient lacking mental capacity to make decisions, DNACPR decision can be made for these patients if it is believed to be in their best interests. However before making this decision, the following need to be performed -
Check for any advance directives,
Discussion with individual with lasting power of attorney or an Independent mental capacity advocate. Discuss with next of kin/close relatives to explore patient's beliefs and wishes.
Refer to local hospital guidelines.
Senior clinicians/Consultants will need to be involved in this process.

In case of emergency, it will be impossible to perform above checks. In such situation decision lies with the treating Consultant.
(DNACPR decisions who decides and how? National End of Life Care Programme, NHS - http://www.lwdwtraining.uk/wp-content/uploads/2012/09/DNACPR-decisions-who-decides-and-how-Sept-2012.pdf)

Mental capacity act 2005
(www.legislation.gov.uk):

The principles:
A person must be assumed to have capacity unless it is established that he/she lacks capacity.

A person is not to be treated as unable to make a decision unless all practicable steps to help him/her to do so have been taken without success.

A person is not to be treated as unable to make a decision merely because he/she makes an unwise decision.

An act done, or decision made, under this Act for or on behalf of a person who lacks capacity must be done, or made, in his/her best interests.

Before the act is done, or the decision is made, regard must be had to whether the purpose for which it is needed can be as effectively achieved in a way that is less restrictive of the person's rights and freedom of action.

How is mental capacity determined?

Mental capacity act suggests that a patient is unable to make decision if they cannot
1. Understand the information relevant to the decision

2. Retain that information
3. Use or weigh up that information as part of the process of making the decision

Most Hospitals have a 'Mental Capacity Assessment Tool' for assessment. (You will need to familiarise with the one in your hospital)

Scenario 4. Telephone conversation: You are the on call registrar. You have seen an open femoral fracture in A&E sustained following RTC and you will need to discuss this with your on call consultant. The open wound measures about 1cm, appears clean. Pulse rate – 110/min, BP 100/70 mmhg, RR – 18/min.
This question will assess your approach to major trauma, trauma management and communication skills.

Using structure 'UR TABLE PC' as follows:

U – ATLS station
R – Telephone conversation role

T – Communicate over phone (As mentioned previously, when discussing about patients with colleagues or seniors, *SBAR protocol is useful)
A –Confirm you have done everything right and if there is anything else to be done with the Consultant (You should have done the initial

management already before speaking to the consultant, remember you are the registrar on call).
B – be confident.
L – Listen to any questions/answer appropriately.
E – Show empathy by acknowledging the seriousness of the injury.

P – Make a plan before discussing with consultant
C – Be clear

This is ATLS scenario. Before discussing with your consultant make up a management plan based on ATLS guidelines. If there is a paper provided, make a quick note.
Applying ATLS principles to this question
C spine immobilized,
A – Airway management with C Spine control: Airway clear as patient talking, start high flow oxygen, C Spine immobilised
B – Breathing: Good bilateral symmetrical chest expansion, Normal resonance on percussion, normal breath sounds, trachea central, respiratory rate 16, oxygen saturations 99%.
C – Circulation with Haemorrhage control: Tachycardia with low BP, patient in grade 2 hypotensive shock. Examine the four sources of blood loss – chest, abdomen, pelvis, long bones. In this scenario with isolated loManagement - Two wide bore cannula, one in each arm, bloods sent for fbc, u&E, lactate, 4 units cross match. One litre Hartmann fluids started in each arm. Arterial blood

gas and catheterization performed provided no bruising in perineal region.
D – Glasgow coma score and pupils symmetrical,
E - Exposure – Deformed femur. Wound at femur fracture site is clean, no extravasation. Photograph taken, saline soaked gauze, analgesia, antibiotics, tetanus cover, Thomas splint. Reassess circulation, if not responding transfuse blood products. Usually do not require to activate major haemorrhage pathway for isolated femur fracture. However you will need to be aware of the major haemorrhage protocol in your hospital. (Should know BOAST guidelines for open fractures www.boa.ac.uk).

Also if injury happened in daytime, as part of your plan prepare patient for theatre. Therefore you should know when the patient last ate and drank, discuss with theatre co ordinator, trauma theatre staff, anaesthetist, radiographers, plastic surgery colleagues. If patient arrives at night, generally can wait till morning for surgery, if stable.

KNOW your ATLS – This will recur in clinical station as well

SBAR protocol to be used while informing about patient to Consultant:
S – Situation
Introduce yourself, check you are speaking to the correct person, inform patient details.
B – Background
Mode of injury, any past medical history.

A – Assessment
Your assessment of patient. ATLS type description – ABCDE. Investigations. Also mention any relevant patient concerns. (In this scenario, you are concerned that the patient is in hypovolemic shock, however you have started treatment to stabilize this)
R – Remedy
Your management plan being discussed with Consultant. IV fluids, cross match, bloods, analgesia, antibiotics, photograph, dressing, Thomas splint. Discuss with theatre co ordinator, trauma theatre staff, anaesthetist, radiographers, plastic surgery colleagues. If patient arrives at night, generally can wait till morning for surgery, if stable and wound satisfactory (Read BOAST guidelines www.boa.ac.uk).

Scenario 5. Consent scenarios:
5A. You are the registrar on call and have been asked to consent a 40 year old patient admitted earlier in the day with an undisplaced intracapsular fracture neck of femur sustained following RTC, for whom a Dynamic Hip Screw fixation has been planned.

Apply principles of UR TABLE PC

U – It is about consenting
R – Get into the role of the operating Surgeon

T – You will need to discuss about benefits and possible complications of DHS for intracapsular fracture neck of femur.
A – Ask if patient has any questions, if everything was clear
B – Confident, eye to eye contact
L – Patient will have questions, so listen and answer appropriately
E – Understand patient's concerns, especially as you would have mentioned about the risk of Avascular Necrosis and other complications.

P – Know when the surgery would be performed approximately. Also need to mention about post operative plan, time off work etc... Also will need to mention about potentially requiring either an open reduction or conversion to total hip replacement, depending on the fracture configuration and displacement when screened in theatre under image intensifier.

While consenting patients, you should be aware of why the procedure is carried out, are there any other alternatives, what does the procedure actually involve, benefits, post operative plan including expected outcomes and follow up, what are the potential complications
One way to ensure all the relevant details are mentioned while consenting patients for any procedure, is to add P before ABC = PA PB PC

P – Purpose the procedure is done/Why is this procedure being done.
A – Alternative procedures if available
P – Procedure itself
B – Benefits
P – Post operative plan including follow up
C - Complications

5B. Mr.David had tibial nailing performed yesterday evening. This morning he woke up with severe pain and compartment syndrome is suspected. Emergency fasciotomy has been arranged. You will need to consent this patient.

These 2 stations are about consent. You can be asked to consent for hip hemiarthroplasty, DHS, distal radius plating, THR, TKR, fasciotomy, supracondylar fracture fixation in children.
Follow 'PA PB PC' protocol so that you cover all the relevant details.
P – Purpose the procedure is done/Why is this procedure being done.
A – Alternative procedures if available
P – Procedure itself
B – Benefits
P – Post operative plan including follow up
C - Complications

General complications for any surgery include infection, bleeding, stiffness, damage to

surrounding nerves and blood vessels, re surgery, scar tenderness.
In addition, for joint replacements mention about implant complications such as dislocation, fracture, wear, loosening, leg length discrepancy. For fasciotomy also mention that the wounds will be reassessed and good chance they will need skin grafting under care of plastic surgeons. For fracture fixation also mention about failure of fixation, redisplacement.
Consent stations can also assess your clinical knowledge, although strictly speaking this is a communication station. The patient in the above example might ask about compartment syndrome, its causes, treatments etc........This is covered in clinical stations.

Scenario 6. You have performed distal radius plating for fracture on 32 year old Ms.Anne. However during surgery radial artery was accidently incised and had to be ligated. You are seeing Ms.Anne in post surgery ward round.

UR TABLE PC

U –This station is about being genuine and honest.
R – Get into the role of Surgeon.

T – Communicate with actor

A – Ask questions as to whether she is comfortable post op, sickness settling, move fingers checking for neurological status, check perfusion
B – Confident, eye to eye contact
L – Listen to patient queries. Patient bound to ask 'How did the operation go doctor?'
E – Empathise with post operative pain if there is. Reassure the patient. Explain about radial artery ligation. Empathise with her concerns, but reassure that ulnar artery was tested intraoperatively (Allens test) and was intact. This should be sufficient to perfuse hand and fracture should heal well. Although the swelling can take a bit longer than usual to settle.

P – Plan to reassess again before discharge. Keep overnight to assess hand perfusion. Explain post operative rehabilitation plan. Plaster for 2 weeks, fracture clinic review in 2 weeks, no load bearing on arm for 6 weeks atleast.
C- Ask if there are any more questions.

Presentation and list planning

Presentation station: Topic provided few weeks before presentation. Presentation is for about 3 minutes (check applicant handbook, as this can change).
Keep the presentation smart. Do not overfill the slide with words/sentences. Use pictures where possible to explain or represent things. Remember your Interviewer has been listening to the same presentation all day. Have bullet points, do not overfill with sentences. Make it legible and easy to read, while you are talking.

Practice your presentation to maintain time. Start with brief topic introduction, progress rapidly to the main topic and finish with summary/conclusion. Most importantly maintain your time. Likely to score higher for finishing on time. For example, you could keep 30 seconds for introduction, 2 minutes for the main topic and 30 seconds for summary or conclusion.

It is difficult to present all information in 3 minutes, this station will assess your organisation skills, time management and communication. Quote literature evidence if available to demonstrate evidence based practice. As the topic is usually provided few weeks in advance, you will have sufficient time to practice. Be prepared for some questioning about the topic. For example, if asked to present about

“Future of orthopaedics”, Consider demonstrating future training, future research, robotic surgery etc.

List planning:

National Confidential Enquiry into Patient Outcome and Death (NCEPOD) Classification of Intervention (WWW.NCEPOD.ORG.UK)

(NCEPOD 1)IMMEDIATE – Immediate life, limb or organ-saving. Normally within minutes of decision to operate.
(NCEPOD 2) URGENT – Intervention for acute onset or clinical deterioration of potentially life or limb threatening conditions, for fixation of many fractures, for relief of pain or other distressing symptoms. Normally within hours of decision to operate.

(NCEPOD 3)EXPEDITED – Patient requiring early treatment where the condition is not an immediate threat to life, limb or organ survival. Normally within days of decision to operate.

(NCEPOD 4)ELECTIVE – Intervention planned or booked in advance of routine admission to hospital. Timing to suit patient, hospital and staff.

List priorities:

- Life and limb threatening injuries (NCEPOD 1) need to go ASAP – compartment syndrome, fracture with significant vascular injury, septic patients. They cannot wait till next morning.
- Fractures depending on the severity can wait till morning. It will be your judgement to decide if they need to go first on the list. Example – open fracture with intact vascularity/pulse.
- Latex allergy – The entire theatre needs to be cleared of any latex items, this will require time. To avoid unnecessary delay between surgeries, prioritise them first on the list if possible, AM or PM list
- Paediatric patient – Kids require priority, as they do not tolerate being fasted all day very well.
- Most hospitals have local policies for prioritising patients. Familiarise with your hospital policy.

Aim of prioritising surgical patients for theatre:
To minimise harm to patients.
To optimise use of theatre time.
To minimise delays.
To minimise avoidable cancellations

Theatre co-ordinator, waiting list co ordinator, booking clerks are essential key players.

There is no right or wrong answer while prioritising lists. As long as you are able to justify your priorities, you will be fine.
Often scenarios will have similarly urgent cases requiring surgery. As long as you can logically discuss and justify your list priorities, you will be fine.
Don't forget, you can also mention about discussing with theatre co-ordinator to see if there is any spare/extra theatre space available.
Useful to know approximate timing for each operation including anaesthetic time, as theatre time can be optimised adequately.
When mentioning about lunch break, say that the break time is flexible depending on how the list is making progress.

PAIR protocol can be used to prioritise patients on theatre list.
Essentially PAIR stands for
P – Priorities: Which patients need to be prioritised.
A – Availability: What are the available resources.
I – Impediments: what are the impediments/obstacles for prioritising patients.
R- Remedy – Final list.

'PAIR' protocol

Priorities NCEPOD classification, Latex allergy pts, Paediatric patients, Daycase patients to allow early discharge, Patients with diabetes, Frail patients, ASA 3 or more, Surgery for infection usually at end of list if systemically well.	Availability Paediatric anaesthetists for paediatric cases, HDU/ICU bed availability if patient unwell pre operatively, Combined case – appropriate teams availability, Extra theatre availability (emergency theatre for any emergency cases). Appropriate implants availability, Image intensifier availability.
Impediments Blood results – high INR, low Haemoglbin etc… Theatre time Not notifying wards of the "Golden" patient (patient to go first on the list)	Remedy Optimise List planning skills

Examples:

Q1. You are the trauma registrar and have been asked to make an order of the list by your Consultant, who will be arriving 10 minutes late. It is a full day trauma theatre.

OR

Instead of planning the list directly, you could be asked to discuss with the SHO on call regarding patients awaiting theatre and then to inform the Consultant on call regarding the list you have planned for next morning. Essentially principles remain the same.

1. 6 year old with grade 2 supracondylar right elbow fracture for MUA + k wire
2. 80 year old left intracapsular neck of femur fracture with latex allergy for hemiarthroplasty
3. Grade 2 open left tibia fracture for debridement + IM nail
4. Right big toe abscess for incision and drainage
5. Right distal radius fracture for ORIF
6. Right Weber B ankle fracture for ORIF

Answer:
Before you make an order, need to gather more information using 'PAIR' protocol.

P (Priorities) –
Patient 1 is paediatric
Patient 2 has latex allergy
Patient 3 has compound fracture

Find out if Patient 4 is systemically well.
Find out if Patient 6 has any ankle subluxation/dislocation.

A (Availability) –
Is Image intensifier available for the full list
Is the trauma anaesthetist able to anaesthetize paediatric patient 1
What time does the list start and finish (if not mentioned in the question)
Is a plastic surgeon available to look at open tibia wound

I (Impediments) –
The theatre time available is not sufficient to perform all operations. So if there is a slot available in emergency theatre, can the toe abscess be drained in emergency theatre.
Also make sure blood results for all the patients are satisfactory.
Make sure ankle is not too swollen to operate (Patient 6).

R (Remedy) – List planning
(N.B – The following order is not the only order possible. You can form the list in any order as long as you can substantiate your order with a logical thinking process. Expected operating time including anaesthetic time in brackets next to the procedure)
My order of the list will be:

1. Right supracondylar elbow fracture – MUA +/- k wire (45 minutes, need image intensifier)
2. Left Open tibia fracture – Wound debridement + IM nailing (120 minutes, need image intensifier)
Lunch break
3. Left Hip hemiarthroplasty (90 minutes)
4. Right Ankle ORIF (60 minutes, need image intensifier)
5. Right Big toe abscess Incision and Drainage (40 minutes)

Unfortunately I will need to cancel patient with distal radius fracture, due to lack of theatre space. I will consider Paediatric supracondylar fracture patient at top of my list as patient is a child, also if left too long, it can be difficult to reduce the fracture closed and also there is risk of compartment syndrome.
Open tibia fracture will be second on my list has the wound needs to be debrided ASAP to decrease risk of infection and also provide soft tissues to heal. Also plastic surgeons suggested they were available in the morning to review the wound in theatre.
Lunch break will provide time for theatres to be prepared to allow surgery on latex allergy neck of femur fracture patient.
I have considered Ankle fracture over distal radius as ankles have a tendency to swell and can delay surgery if not operated on early.
Abscess patient is last as it is infected case and also patient is systemically well and therefore can wait till end of the list.

I will warn patient with ankle fracture, that there is a potential for cancellation, if we run out of theatre time, as I will then need to prioritise toe abscess patient over ankle fracture. This is to prevent abscess patient form becoming systemically unwell.

Q2. You have been asked to plan elective list by your consultant who would like to assess your list planning skills. The elective list runs from 8Am to 5PM. Image intensifier is only available in the afternoon.
1. 50 year old gentleman with type 2 diabetes for right carpal tunnel decompression under LA
2. 6 year old boy for removal of tens nail from left femur
3. 78 year old type 2 diabetic for right total hip replacement
4. Exchange nailing for infected non union of left tibia in a 36 year old
5. 80 year old for right total knee replacement

Answer:
PAIR protocol
P (Priorities) –
Paediatric patient for removal of nail.
Diabetic patient for hip replacement.
Day case surgery patients - carpal tunnel decompression and removal of tens nail.

A (Availability)
Image intensifier available in afternoon only. Therefore exchange nailing will need to be performed in the afternoon.
For Removal of tens nail, image intensifier is not necessary as the nails were palpable subcutaneously, when assessed in clinic. However this will be reassessed on day of surgery. (Need to ask interviewer whether nail ends are easily palpable. If buried in bone, might need to have image intensifier available)

I (Impediment)
Image intensifier available in afternoon only.
Make sure blood results are satisfactory for all patients.

R (Remedy)
1. Right Carpal tunnel decompression (15 minutes). This is first since it is day case procedure and under Local Anaesthesia.
2. Right total hip replacement (120 minutes). As this patient has diabetes, I would not like to starve this patient for long hours.
3. Right total knee replacement (120 minutes).
Lunch break
4. Left femur – Removal of TENS nail (45 minutes). Paediatric patient for removal of nail will be first on the afternoon list (If nail ends are buried). This is because, we might require image intensifier and this is available in the afternoon only. (If the nail

ends are palpable, could consider doing this patient 3rd on the list and change knee replacement to 4th)
5. Left tibia Exchange IM nailing (120 minutes). This is last since it requires image intensifier and is infected

Q3. You are the trauma registrar delegated to plan trauma list for the full day. Consultant is also in theatre.
1. Grade 3 supracondylar left elbow fracture in 5 year old.
2. Grade 2 open right tibia in 20 year old for wound debridement + External fixator
3. 40 year old with intracapsular left neck of femur fracture for Cannulated screw fixation
4. 80 year old type 2 diabetic with left intertrochanteric fracture for DHS
5. 30 year old latex allergy patient with right ankle fracture for Ankle ORIF

Answer:
PAIR protocol
P (Priorities)
Grade 3 supracondylar as it can lead to neurovascular compromise and also can be difficult to perform closed reduction if not dealt with ASAP.
Compound tibia fracture patient due to increased risk of bone infection if fractures and wound not dealt with. Plastic surgeons will also be required in theatre to assess wound.

40 year old with intracapsular neck of femur needs to be fixed ASAP to minimize risk of AVN of femoral head.
Diabetic patient with neck of femur needs to be prioritized as well.

A (Availability)
Check theatre start and finish times, if not mentioned.
Image intensifier is needed for the full list.

I (Impediment)
Latex allergy patient will require theatre preparation before surgery.
Make sure blood results are satisfactory for all patients.

R (Remedy) My list-
Start your answer by saying, this is a complex situation. This shows the interviewer that you have understood the gravity of the current situation. The first 3 cases on the list need to be dealt with ASAP.As there is only one theatre list available, they will need to be sequenced and therefore, they may all not get the top spot.
I will keep the same order as mentioned in the question.
1. Left Supracondylar elbow fracture MUA + K Wire +/- Open reduction (45 minutes)
2. Right Open tibia fracture – wound debridement + temporary external fixator (60 minutes)
3. Left Hip Cannulated screw fixation (60 minutes)

Lunch break
4. Left Hip DHS (60 minutes)
5. Right Ankle ORIF (60 minutes)

Child with grade 3 supracondylar needs to be reduced ASAP to minimize neurovascular compromise and hence will remain on top of my list. Compound fracture needs debridement ASAP and therefore second on my list. Intracapsular neck of femur fracture also needs to be dealt with ASAP, however due to lack of theatre space he will remain third (Debatable, can be pushed second, but as mentioned, you should be able to justify your answer).
I appreciate we have a diabetic patient on the list, but however patient will need to wait and will remain fourth on the list. He can have early breakfast. Also, I will ensure ward staff measure BMs regularly while fasted as per Hospital protocol. The last patient has latex allergy and therefore there will be some delay between cases. I would have informed patient in the morning that if time does not permit, we might have to cancel surgery on that particular day and try to perform that patient first on the next day's list.

To demonstrate lateral thinking process, you could also mention:
I will discuss with theatre co-ordinator to see if there is any other theatre space available. Also will check if there is another surgeon and image intensifier available. My Consultant will be supervising me. If

available one of the patients can be transferred to that extra list

(N.B – Some scenarios are difficult to prioritise one above another as they can all be of similar complexity and emergency. But the idea with these stations is to assess your approach to list planning and rationale thinking. So it does not matter, which cases are on top of the list as long as it is supported by a good decision making process)

Q4. You are requested to organise Mr.M's elective list. The list includes
1. Right shoulder replacement in a 70 year. Previously cancelled once.
2. Right shoulder arthroscopic subacromial decompression in a 50 year old.
3. Right midshaft humerus non union ORIF in a 65 year old. Patient is ASA 4.
4. Right carpal tunnel decompression under LA.

Answer:
PAIR protocol
P (Priorities)
Patient for shoulder replacement cancelled previously.
Patient for midshaft humerus fracture is ASA 4.
Carpal tunnel decompression patient is day case.

A (Availability)
Image intensifier for midshaft humerus non union will be required.
The same patient is ASA 4 and will need to discuss with anesthetist regarding need for post op HDU care and bed availability.

I (Impediment)
IF HDU bed is required for Midshaft humerus non union patient, this is to be checked before surgery. If no beds available, surgery might need to be cancelled.
Make sure blood results are satisfactory for all patients.

R (Remedy)
1. Right Carpal tunnel decompression (15 minutes) under LA, as the procedure is quick and day case.
2. Right Midshaft humerus non union ORIF (120 minutes). This patient is ASA 4 and might need HDU care post op. So better done early in the day.
Lunch break
3.Right Shoulder replacement (120 minutes). I will not want this patient to wait till the very end , as the patient has already been cancelled once.
4.Right shoulder subacromial decompression (60 minutes).

Q5. You are requested to lead the morning trauma meeting (Lucky you). This also requires organising the theatre list. The list includes:
1.Right distal radius fracture in a 50 year old for ORIF. Previously cancelled twice.
2. 60 year old with left ankle fracture for ORIF. On warfarin for Atrial Fibrillation. INR 2.1
3. 80 year old right hip intracapsular neck of femur fracture for hemiarthroplasty. ASA 4.
4. 30 year old septic patient for washout of infected left knee.
5. 30 year old with right tibia fracture for IM nail.
6. Cauda Equina syndrome patient for L4 discectomy.

Answer:
This is a challenging situation. There are few patients on the list that need to be dealt with ASAP.As there is only one theatre list available, they will need to be sequenced and therefore, they may all not get the top spot.

I will discuss with theatre co-ordinator to see if there is any other theatre space available. Also will check if there is another surgeon is available. My Consultant will be supervising my operating. If available one of the patients (either the septic knee patient or cauda equine syndrome) can be transferred to that extra theatre list, depending on the operating Surgeon's preference and experience and also availability of image intensifier.

P (Priorities) –
Septic patient with knee infection.
Impending cauda equine syndrome patient, as delayed surgery can lead to bladder and bowel incompetence (Read Cauda Equina Syndrome in Clinical section)
Neck of femur patient who is ASA 4.
Distal radius fracture, as patient cancelled twice.

A (Availability) –
Image intensifier for all patient except infected knee.
Will check with anaesthetist if septic patient requires HDU post op.
Also if Neck of femur patient requires HDU post op.

I (Impediment) –
Patient with ankle fracture has INR 2.1. At my hospital the protocol is to operate if the INR is <1.5 (some hospitals at INR<2). Will need Vitamin K for reversal and repeat INR later in the day.
Realistically, if there is only one theatre list, we will not have sufficient time to operate on the ankle fracture and therefore will cancel this patient early in the day, to avoid unnecessary fasting for the patient.

R (Remedy) –
1. Left knee washout (45 – 60 minutes). Septic patient with knee infection, as the patient is septic. This is a life saving procedure. Anaesthesia might require more time than normal, as patient is septic and may require invasive monitoring.
2. Cauda Equina Syndrome patient for L4 discectomy (60 minutes), as this is also an emergency.
3. Right Hip hemiarthroplasty (60 - 90 minutes). Intracapsular neck of femur fracture patient will be third due to ASA. Anaesthesia will be challenging due to ASA, therefore expect some delay.
Lunch break
3. Right distal Radius ORIF (60 minutes). Distal radius fracture will be third, as he was cancelled twice previously.
4. Right Tibia IM nail (90 minutes). Will warn patient earlier in the day that surgery might get cancelled, depending on the time required for earlier surgeries.

Left ankle ORIF will need to be cancelled due to lack of time and high INR. Will add this patient first on next day's trauma list if possible.

Clinical Anatomy stations

Preparation for this station should begin well in advance, ideally few months. As Orthopaedic trainee (at any level) you should have a good understanding of basic musculoskeletal anatomy. The following list is not exhaustive. But you should be thorough with these, as it covers most topics.

Upper Limb:

Median nerve:

Arises from lateral and medial cords of brachial plexus.

Enters axilla at inferior margin of teres major.

It starts lateral to brachial artery and then crosses superficial to the artery to lie on the medial side of the artery in the upper arm. Does not provide any branches in the upper arm.

It enters the elbow between the two heads of pronator teres.

It then travels between flexor digitorum superficialis and flexor digitorum profundus. At the wrist it lies between flexor carpi radialis and palmaris longus. Enters hand through carpal tunnel.

Branches:

Anterior interosseous nerve: Arises in the proximal forearm. Accompanies anterior interosseous artery and supplies flexor pollicics longus, pronator quadratus and lateral half of flexor digitorum profundus (to index and middle fingers).

Palmar Cutaneous branch: Arises proximal to wrist and supplies sensations to thenar eminence.

Recurrent motor branch: arises in hand and supplies opponens pollicis, abductor pollicis brevis and superficial part of flexor pollicis brevis.

Median nerve : Median nerve supplies: FCR, Palmaris longus, FDS, 1st and 2nd lumbricals.

Digital cutaneous branches in hand supply radial three and half digits.

Ulnar Nerve:

Arises from medial cord of brachial plexus.
Descends on postero-medial aspect of humerus.
At the elbow lies posterior to medial epicondyle.
At proximal forearm passes to anterior compartment between 2 heads of Flexor Carpi Ulnaris.
Travels in medial aspect of forearm and lies medial to ulnar artery.
Enters hand through Guyon's canal.
Muscles innervated: FCU, medial half FDP, Medial 2 lumbricals, All interossei

Radial nerve:

Radial nerve arises from posterior cord of brachial plexus.

Enters posterior compartment through triangular interval (bounded by teres major superior, long head triceps medial and humeral shaft lateral).

Lies in spiral groove at posterior surface of humerus and is accompanied by profunda brachii artery.

About 5cm proximal to elbow joint, it enters anterior compartment by piercing lateral intermuscular septum.

It lies anterior to lateral epicondyle and proceeds towards radial head where it divides into a superficial branch (superficial radial nerve) and deep branch (posterior interosseous nerve).

Superficial radial nerve runs underneath brachioradialis. Proximal to the wrist it enters posterior compartment. It supplies sensations to dorsum of first web space.

PIN passes between the 2 heads of supinator and enters posterior compartment to supply all muscles of posterior compartment except Triceps, brachioradialis, ECRL, which are supplied by Radial nerve.

Deltopectoral approach to shoulder:
Patient position – Beach chair
Skin incision – Coracoid process to anterior margin of deltoid.
Internervous plane – Axillary nerve (deltoid) and medial/lateral pectoral nerves (pectoralis major)
Identify cephalic vein.
Gently dissect and retract Cephalic vein lateral with deltoid
Identify coracoid, stay lateral to coracoid (medial to coracoid is danger territory – brachial plexus and axillary artery)
Identify conjoint tendon
Dissect Lateral to conjoint tendon
Onto subscapularis
If fixing proximal humerus fractures, do not need to incise subscapularis. Instead apply stay sutures at supscapularis (lesser tuberosity fragment), and supraspinatus/ teres minor (Greater tuberosity fragment) at this stage. Stay sutures will be used to reduce the tuberosities onto the plate.
If performing arthroplasty - Incise subscapularis about 1- 2 cm from insertion leaving the lower fourth intact (some prefer not to leave the lower portion intact) followed by capsular incision to enter glenohumeral joint.
Structures at risk – stay lateral to coracoid to avoid brachial plexus and axillary vessels

Rotator cuff muscles:

Rotator cuff	Origin	Insertion	Function	Nerve supply
Supraspinatus muscle	supraspinatus fossa	Superior facet Greater Tuberosity	Abduction	Suprascapular nerve
Infraspinatus	Infraspinatus fossa	Mddle facet Greater tuberosity	External Rotation	Suprascapular nerve
Teres Minor	Middle half lateral border	Inferior facet Greater tuberosity	External Rotation	Axillary nerve
Subscapularis	Subscapularis fossa	Lesser Tuberosity	Internal Rotation	Upper and Lower Subscapular nerves

Anterior approach for proximal shaft humerus fractures:

(Anterior approach advantageous for proximal and midshaft fractures, as it can be extended proximally to deltopectoral approach. With posterior approach, proximal extension is limited due to posterior deltoid and axillary nerve)

Patient position – Supine or Beach chair
Skin incision – lateral border of biceps (can be extended proximally to deltopectoral approach if required)
Internervous plane –
Superficial interval between biceps (musculocutaneous nerve) and brachialis (dual nerve supply musculocutaneous and radial nerves).
Deep interval between 2 parts of brachialis - medial half supplied by musculocutaneous and lateral half by radial nerve. This division of nerve supply is not absolute and is variable.
After skin incision, identify lateral border of biceps and retract it medial
Identify brachialis
Split brachialis in middle onto humeral shaft.

Arm Anterior compartment muscles:

Muscle	Origin	Insertion	Action	Nerve supply
Biceps brachii	Long head – supraglenoid tubercle Short head – Coracoid process	Radial tuberosity	Elbow supination Elbow flexion	Musculocutaneous nerve
Brachialis	Distal Anterior shaft humerus	Coronoid process	Elbow flexion	Musculocutaneous and Radial nerves
Coracobrachialis	Coracoid process	Medial mid shaft humerus	Shoulder flexion & adduction	Musculocutaneous nerve

Posterior approach to humerus for lower third humerus fractures:

Patient position – Lateral, arm resting on arm support.
Skin incision – Midline posterior
Internervous plane – Between heads of triceps (all supplied by radial nerve). So no true internervous plane.
Superficial split between long head and lateral head followed by dissection of distal tendon in midline.
Deep split between medial and lateral head.
Neurovascular structures between medial and

lateral head. (neurovascular structures in the spiral groove, if no fractures). This approach is often performed for fractures and anatomy may be altered. Therefore need to palpate neurovascular structures during all phases of dissection, to prevent accidental damage.
Neurovascular structures in spiral groove – Radial nerve and Profunda brachii artery
Structures at risk - Radial nerve and Profunda brachii artery

(For fixation of distal humerus fractures, you will usually remain distal to spiral groove without needing to expose radial nerve. For distal humerus intraarticular fractures, olecranon osteotomy is usually required)

Arm Posterior compartment muscles:

Muscle	Origin	Insertion	Action	Nerve supply
Long head triceps	Infraglenoid tubercle	Olecranon	Elbow extension	Radial nerve
Lateral head triceps	Posterior humerus proximal to spiral groove	Olecranon	Elbow extension	Radial nerve
Medial head triceps	Posterior humerus distal to spiral groove	Olecranon	Elbow extension	Radial nerve

Cubital fossa:
Boundaries:
Superior – Imaginary line connecting medial and lateral epicondyles.
Medial – Lateral border of pronator teres.
Lateral – Medial border of brachioradialis.

Floor consists of Brachialis and supinator muscles. Roof consists of skin, superficial fascia containing the median cubital vein, the lateral cutaneous nerve of the forearm and the medial cutaneous nerve of the forearm, deep fascia reinforced by the bicipital aponeurosis.

Contents
Biceps tendon
Brachial artery: Lies medial to tendon.
Median nerve: Lies medial to brachial artery.
Radial nerve lies laterally between brachioradialis and brachialis.

Volar Henry approach forearm:
Patient position – supine, arm resting on arm table.
Skin incision – lateral border of biceps tendon at elbow to radial styloid at wrist.
(Lateral cutaneous nerve of foream lies superficial to brachioradialis and often encountered in proximal approach.
Superficial radial nerve lies underneath brachioradialis at proximal and middle portions of the approach. Radial artery lies underneath

brachioradialis medial to superficial radial nerve at proximal and middle portions of the approach. Distally it lies medial to brachioradialis)
Need to utilize only the relevant section of the approach.
For ease we will divide this approach into proximal, middle and distal parts.

Proximal volar henry approach:
Internervous plane – brachioradialis (radial nerve) and biceps tendon (musculocutaneous nerve) at elbow. brachioradialis (radial nerve) and pronator teres (median nerve) a bit distally.
Incide deep fascia.
Recurrent radial artery branches (Leash of Henry) need to be ligated to mobilise brachioradialis lateral.
Develop a plane between brachioradialis and biceps tendon/pronator teres.
Keep arm supinated to mobilise posterior interosseous nerve away from the field. Posterior interosseous nerve pierces supinator and enters posterior compartment. Remember, Supination mobilises the nerve more dorsal. Pronation mobilises it more volar.
Identify biceps tendon and dissect lateral to biceps tendon to expose proximal radius. Remember brachial artery s medial to biceps tendon. Supinator will need to be elevated from bone, keeping the arm supinated to expose radius proximally.
Dangers: Posterior interosseous nerve, radial artery, lateral cutaneous nerve forearm.

Middle volar henry approach:
Internervous plane – brachioradialis (radial nerve) and pronator teres (median nerve)
Incise deep fascia.
Develop a plane between brachioradialis and pronator teres.
Pronator teres insertion will need to be elevated to expose mid third radius. Keep arm pronated to elevate pronator teres off its insertion.
Dangers: Radial artery, lateral cutaneous nerve forearm, superficial radial nerve.

Distal volar henry approach:
Internervous plane – Brachioradialis (radial nerve) and Flexor Carpi Radialis (Median nerve).
Dissect between Brachioradialis and FCR. Flexor pollicis longus and Pronator quadratus in deep layers. Retract Flexor pollicis longus (medially or laterally depending on the fracture configuration and fixation). Pronator quadratus incised laterally at radius to expose volar distal radius.
Dangers: Radial artery, median nerve.

Volar forearm muscles:

Remember Common flexor origin – medial epicondyle humerus

Muscle	Origin	Insertion	Action	Nerve supply
Pronator teres	Humeral head - Common flexor origin Ulnar head – coronoid process	Middle third lateral shaft radius	Forearm pronation	Median nerve
Flexor carpi radialis	Common flexor origin	Bases of second and third metacarpals	Wrist flexion Wrist Radial deviation	Median nerve
Palmaris longus	Common flexor origin	Palmar aponeurosis	Wrist flexion	Median nerve
Flexor Carpi Ulnaris	Humeral head - Common flexor origin. Ulnar head – medial olecranon	Pisiform, hook of hamate, base of 5th metacarpal	Wrist flexion Wrist ulnar deviation	Ulnar nerve
Flexor digitorum superficialis	Common flexor origin, Proximal radius and proximal ulna	Bases of middle phalanx 2nd to 5th fingers	PIPJ flexion 2nd to 5th fingers	Median nerve
Flexor	Middle and	Base of	Thumb	Anterior

pollicis longus	Distal radius	distal phalanx Thumb	DIPJ flexion	interosseous nerve
Flexor digitorum Profundus	Proximal and middle ulna, interosseous membrane	Bases of distal phalanx 2nd to 5th fingers	Wrist flexion DIPJ flexion 2nd to 5th fingers	Anterior interosseus nerve, Ulnar nerve
Pronator Quadratus	Distal volar ulna	Distal volar radius	Forearm pronation	Anterior interosseus nerve

Posterior approach Radius/forearm (Thompson approach)

Patient position – supine, arm resting on arm table.
Skin incision – lateral epicondyle elbow to Lister's tubercle radius
Internervous plane- proximally between ECRB (radial nerve) and EDC (Posterior interosseous nerve). Distally between ECRB (radial nerve) and EPL (Posterior interosseous nerve),
In the proximal approach, keep arm pronated, to mobilise posterior interosseous nerve volar.

Extensor wrist compartments:

Compartment	Muscles
1	Abductor pollicis Longus & Extensor pollicis brevis
2	Extensor Carpi Radialis Longus & extensor carpi Radialis brevis
3	Extensor pollicis longus
4	Extensor Indicis & Extensor digitorum communis
5	Extensor digiti minimi
6	Extensor carpi ulnaris

Carpal tunnel decompression:

Carpal tunnel consists of 9 flexor tendons and median nerve.
Flexor retinaculum or Transverse Carpal Ligament attached laterally to scaphoid tuberosity and ridge of trapezium
Medially to pisiform and hook of hamate.
Skin incision – Incision along radial border of ring finger from distal volar wrist crease to Kaplans cardinal line.
Kaplans cardinal line – Imaginary line extending from ulnar border of radially deviated thumb to hook of hamate. Some authors have suggested this line from ulnar border of radially deviated thumb parallel to proximal wrist crease.

Layers from superficial to deep:
Skin
Subcutaneous fat

Palmar aponeurosis/deep fascia (longitudinally oriented fibres)
Flexor retinaculum or Transverse Carpal Ligament (Transversely oriented fibres)

Dangers:
If incision too radial, can injure palmar cutaneous branch of median nerve or even recurrent motor branch of median nerve.
Recurrent motor branch of median nerve has a variable course – can either pass deep to flexor retinaculum (subligamentous), penetrate flexor retinaculum (transligamentous) or pass superficial to flexor retinaculum (extraligamentous).
If incision too ulnar can encounter ulnar artery or guyons canal.

Forearm fasciotomy:
Volar side – Use Henry approach and carpal tunnel decompression.
2 forearm compartments, superficial and deep. Also need to perform carpal tunnel decompression to minimize median nerve injury.
Can use a separate incision for carpal tunnel decompression.
Some tend to use a single incision – henry approach with a ulnar sided curve at the wrist to join incision for carpal tunnel decompression, obviously need to look out for palmar cutaneous branch of median nerve.

While decompressing forearm compartments, deep layer consists of Flexor Pollicis Longus, Pronator quadratus, Flexor digitorum profundus. So visualisation of these muscles will ensure decompression of deep compartment.

Dorsal side – single compartment. Use Thompson's approach.

Lower limb

Approaches to hip:

Anterior approach hip (Smith Peterson):
Patient position: Supine
Internervous plane –
Superficial - Sartorius (Femoral nerve) and Tensor Fascia lata (Superior gluteal nerve)
Deep – Rectus femoris (Femoral nerve) and Gluteus medius (Superior gluteal nerve)
Skin incision – Along anterior half of iliac crest till ASIS and then curve inferiorly in direction of lateral patella.
Superficial dissection between Sartorius and tensor fascia lata.
Deep dissection between rectus femoris and gluteus medius.
Detach reflected head of rectus femoris from origin at acetabulum.
Externally rotate the hip to stretch capsule followed by capsular incision.

Externally rotate to dislocate the hip.

Structures at risk – lateral cutaneous nerve of thigh superficially and ascending branch of lateral femoral circumflex artery between Sartorius and tensor fascia lata.
Femoral nerve and artery will be medial to Sartorius.

Anterolateral approach hip (Watson Jones):
Patient position: supine
Internervous plane – No true intenervous plane.
Tensor fascia lata (Superior gluteal nerve) and gluteus medius (superior gluteal nerve)
Skin incision – Adduct the leg to make greater trochanter more prominent. 10 – 15 cm longitudinal incision centered at the middle third of greater trochanter, along femoral shaft.
Incise fascia lata along line of skin incision.
Retract fascia lata anteriorly and gluteus medius posteriorly.
Dissect between fascia lata and gluteus medius to reach joint capsule.
Incise capsule.

Lateral approach hip (Hardinge):
Patent position – Supine or Lateral (Original Hardinge approach described with Patient supine)
Incision- Start 5cm proximal to greater trochanter and extend distally centering at tip of trochanter and along shaft of femur. The proximal part of the

incision will have a slight posterior curve. Total length of incision will be between 10 – 15 cm.
Dissect subcutaneous tissue, incise fascia lata along line of skin incision.
Internervous plane – no true internervous plane.
Split gluteus medius (superior gluteal nerve) and vastus lateralis (femoral nerve) in the plane of fibres.
Develop anterior flap consisting of gluteus medius proximally and vastus lateralis distally.
Retain posterior half to two thirds of gluteus medius attachment to greater trochanter.
Split gluteus minimus in the same plane as medius to develop anterior flap.
Capsule incision – T, H shapes described.
Dislocate hip with external rotation.

Danger- Do not split gluteus medius more than 5cm proximal from its insertion, to avoid injury to superior gluteal nerve as it runs between medius and minimus.

Posterior approach hip:
Position – lateral
Skin incision – 10 to 15 cm centred at tip of greater trochanter extending distally along shaft of femur and proximal curve posteriorly in direction of gluteus maximus fibres.
Internervous plane – no true internervous plane.
Incise fascia lata and split gluteus maximus along line of incision

Identify external rotators (piriformis, superior gemellus, obturator internus, inferior gemellus, quadratus femoris)
Incise external rotators at their insertion on femur.
Incise capsule
Internally rotate and dislocate femoral head.

Dangers – Sciatic nerve. It exits pelvis through the greater sciatic foramen and enters posterior thigh inferior to piriformis. Injured by posterior retractors, post operative haematoma.
Anterior retractors can injure femoral nerve, femoral vessels.

Hip external rotators noticed during posterior approach:

Muscle	Origin	Insertion	Action	Nerve supply (All are direct branches from lumbosacral plexus)
Piriformis	Anterior sacral surface	Piriformis fossa medial to greater trochanter	Hip External Rotation	Nerve to piriformis
Superior gemellus	Ischial spine	Upper part of Obturator internus		Nerve to Obturator internus
Obturator Internus	Medial surface of obturator membrane and	Medial greater trochanter		Nerve to obturator internus

	surrounding bone			
Inferior gemellus	Above ischial tuberosity	Lower part of obturator internus		Nerve to quadratus femoris
Quadratus femoris	Ischial tuberosity	Intertrochanteric crest		Nerve to quadratus femoris

Gluteal Muscles:

Muscle	Origin	Insertion	Action	Nerve supply
Gluteus maximus	Posterior gluteal line, iliac crest posterior to this line, posterior sacrum and coccyx	Gluteal tuberosity femur and iliotibial tract	Hip extension and external rotation	Inferior gluteal nerve
Gluteus medius	Ilium between posterior and anterior gluteal lines	Greater trochanter	Hip abduction	Superior gluteal nerve
Gluteus minimus	Ilium between anterior and inferior gluteal lines	Greater trochanter	Hip abduction	Superior gluteal nerve

Tensor fascia lata	Iliac crest including ASIS	Iliotibial tract (Iliotibial tract is inserted on Gerdy's tubercle)	Hip abduction, external rotation, flexion	Superior Gluteal nerve

Blood supply to femoral head:

Profunda femoris artery (branch of femoral artery) gives off medial femoral circumflex artery (MFCA) and lateral femoral circumflex artery (LFCA). MFCA is the main supply and runs posterior and LFCA runs anterior. They form an extracapsular arterial ring which inturn send ascending cervical/retinacular arteries which ascend the neck along the synovium to supply femoral head. The extracapsular ring also provides metaphyseal arterial branches and epiphyseal arterial branches. Obturator artery gives branches within the ligamentum teres which provides a minor supply to the head in adults.

Branches from superior gluteal artery, inferior gluteal artery, MFCA, LFCA form a “Trochanteric Anastomosis” around greater trochanter and also send branches to femoral head along the ascending cervical branches.

Thigh Anterior compartment muscles:

Muscle	Origin	Insertion	Action	Nerve supply
Rectus femoris	Straight head – Anterior inferior Iliac Spine. Reflected head – Superior acetabulum	All four muscles together form Quadriceps tendon inserting on patella tendon	Knee extension, Hip flexion	Femoral nerve
Vastus medialis	Medial femur. Starts at intertrochanteric line extends along pectineal line, medial part of linea aspera and medial supracondylar line		Knee extension	
Vastus Intermedius	Anterior and lateral femur in upper two thirds		Knee extension	
Vastus Lateralis	Lateral femur. Starts at greater trochanter, intertrochanteric line, lateral part of linea aspera		Knee extension	
Sartorius (Largest muscle in the body)	Anterior Superior Iliac Spine	Proximal anteromedial tibia, forming	Flexion and lateral rotation	

		part of Pes Anserinus	of hip. Knee flexion.	

Thigh Medial compartment muscles:

Muscle	Origin	Insertion	Action	Nerve supply
Gracilis	Inferior border of pubic symphysis and inferior pubic ramus	Proximal anteromedial tibia, forming part of Pes Anserinus	Hip - Flexion, internal rotation, adduction. Knee flexion.	Anterior branch of obturator nerve
Pectineus	Pectineal line of pubis at superior pubic ramus	Pectineal line of femur at medial femur	Hip flexion and adduction	Femoral nerve
Adductor Longus	Superior pubic ramus	Middle third linea aspera	Hip Adduction	Anterior branch of obturator nerve
Adductor Brevis	Superior and Inferior pubic ramus	Line extending fro lesser trochanter to linea aspera (upper third)	Hip adduction	Anterior and posterior branches of obturator nerve
Adductor Magnus	Adductor part - Inferior pubic ramus.	Adductor part – Greater trochanter to Linea	Adductor part – Hip Adduction. Hamstrin	Adductor part – Posterior branch of obturator

	Hamstring part – Ischial tuberosity.	aspera. Hamstring part – Linea aspera and adductor tubercle	g part – Hip Extension.	nerve. Hamstring part – Tibial part of sciatic nerve

Thigh Posterior compartment muscles:

Muscle	Origin	Insertion	Action	Nerve supply
Biceps femoris	Long head – Ischial tuberosity. Short head – lateral lip linea aspera	Fibula head	Knee flexion. Hip extension.	Long head – Tibial part of sciatic nerve. Short head – Peroneal part of sciatic nerve.
Semitendinosus	Ischial tuberosity	Proximal anteromedial tibia, forming part of Pes Anserinus	Knee flexion. Hip extension.	Sciatic nerve
Semimembranosus	Ischial tuberosity	Proximal medial tibia	Knee flexion. Hip extension.	Tibial part of sciatic nerve

Remember Pes Anserinus is formed by Sartorius, Gracilis and Semitendinosus.

Distal femur approach for lateral plating:
Longitudinal insion along lateral mid femoral region.
Dissect Subcutaneous tissues in same plane.
Incise Iliotibial band in same plane.
Elevate vastus lateralis of lateral intermuscular septum at proximal part of approach and retract anterior. Distally, there is not much of muscle tissue.

Medial parapatellar approach for Total knee replacement:
Patient position: Supine
Internervous plane – no true internervous plane.
Longitudinal midline incision extending 5cm above patella till tibial tubercle.
Incise through Subcutaneous fat and create a medial flap to expose quadriceps tendon, medial para patellar region and patella tendon.
Incise Quadriceps tendon proximally along medial edge extending in the medial para patellar region and then extending medial to patella tendon.
Medial capsule (deep MCL) usually elevated off bone.
Evert patella and flex knee.

Popliteal fossa:

Boundries

Supero-Medial: Semimembranosus
Supero-Lateral: Biceps femoris
Infero-Medial: Medial head of Gastrocnemius
Infero-Lateral: Lateral Head of Gastrocnemius

Contents:

Popliteal artery. (Artery deepest, followed by vein and nerve. So deep to superficial remember as 'AVN')
Popliteal vein.
Tibial nerve.
Small saphenous vein drains into popliteal vein.
Common peroneal nerve laterally

Sciatic nerve course:

Arises from lumbosacral plexus (L4 – S3).
Exits pelvis through greater sciatic notch inferior to piriformis.
Travels in posterior compartment of thigh behind adductor magnus.
Before entering popliteal fossa divides into tibial nerve which supplies posterior compartment and common peroneal nerve which supplies anterior and lateral compartments of lower leg.

Lower leg muscles:

Anterior compartment:

Muscle	Origin	Insertion	Function	Nerve supply
Tibialis Anterior	Lateral surface proximal tibia	Dorsum Base of 1st metatarsal and medial cuneiform	Ankle dorsiflexion	Deep Peroneal nerve
Extensor Digitorum Longus	Lateral surface tibia, anterior surface interosseous membrane, anterior surface Fibula	Dorsal surface middle and distal phalanges 2nd – 5th toe	2nd – 5th toe dorsiflexion, Ankle dorsiflexion	Deep Peroneal nerve
Extensor hallucis Longus	Mid fibula, interosseous membrane	Big toe base of distal phalanx dorsum	1st toe Dorsiflexion	Deep Peroneal nerve
Peroneus Tertius	Distal Fibula, interosseous membrane	Dorsal surface base of 5th metatarsal	Ankle dorsiflexion	Deep Peroneal nerve

Superficial Posterior compartment:

Gastronemius	Medial head – posterior medial condyle femur, lateral head – posterior lateral condyle femur	Posterior surface Calcaneus via Tendoachilles	Ankle plantarflexion, Knee flexion	Tibial nerve
Soleus	Posterior fibula, middle third medial border and soleal line posterior tibia	Posterior surface Calcaneus via Tendoachilles	Ankle plantarflexion	Tibial nerve
Plantaris	Inferior end lateral supracondylar ridge femur	Medial side of Tendoachilles	Ankle plantarflexion	Tibial nerve

Deep Posterior compartment:

Tibialis posterior	Posterior Tibia, interosseous membrane, posterior fibula	(wide attachment, mainly navicular) Navicular tuberosity, medial cuneiform, cuboid, sustentaculu	Inversion, plantar flexion	Tibial nerve

		m tali, 2nd - 4th metatarsal base		
Flexor Hallucis Longus	Posterior distal fibula, interosseous membrane	Base of distal phalanx 1st toe	1st toe plantarflexion, weak ankle plantarflexion	Tibial nerve
Flexor Digitorum longus	Posterior Tibia	Base of distal phalanx 2nd – 5th toes	2nd – 5th toes plantarflexion, weak ankle plantarflexion	Tibial nerve
Popliteus	Lateral condyle femur, lateral meniscus	Posterior proximal tibia above soleal line	Internally rotates tibia to unlock knee. If tibia fixed on ground, will externally rotate femur.	Tibial nerve

Peroneal compartment (Lateral compartment):

Peroneus Longus	Proximal and middle thirds lateral Fibula	Base of 1st metatarsal and medial cuneiform plantar aspect	1st metatarsal plantar flexion, Ankle plantarflexion	Superficial peroneal nerve
Peroneus Brevis	Middle and distal	Base of 5th metatarsa	Ankle eversion	Superficial peroneal nerve

	thirds lateral Fibula	l lateral aspect		

Fasciotomy lower leg:
Patient position – supine
2 incision technique
Posteromedial incision – 2cm posterior to medial border of tibia. Split fascia over soleus (superficial posterior compartment). Elevate soleus off posterior tibia and proceed laterally on posterior tibial surface to find fascia covering flexor halluces longs (deep posterior compartment). Perform fasciotomy to decompress the deep posterior compartment.

Lateral incision – 2cm anterior to fibula. Identify intermuscular septum and fascia covering anterior compartment and fascia covering lateral compartment. Perform fasciotomy of anterior and lateral compartments.

Skin is not closed following fasciotomy due to swelling. After 48 hours, a second look is performed to assess viability of soft tissue. Perform a delayed primary skin closure, once swelling subsides. If skin closure not possible within 5 – 7 days, consider split thickness skin grafting.

Anterolateral proximal tibia approach for tibial plateau fracture:
Straight or Hockey stick anterolateral incision starting proximal to knee joint line and extending to lateral part of tibial tubercle..
Elevate Tibialis anterior from anterior surface of proximal tibia.
Need to elevate lateral meniscus to assess articular surface.

Medial approach to distal tibia:
More commonly used for ORIF distal tibia.
Skin Incision: start 5 – 7 cm above medial malleolus. Longitudinal incision along mid tibial surface medially or curve distal end anterior at medial surface distal tibia (Watch out for saphenous vein).
Incise subcutaneous tissue in same plane as skin incision, to reach tibial surface.

Anterolateral approach distal tibia:
Skin incision: Longitudinal incision over anterior edge of fibula.
Internervous plane: Peroneus brevis (superficial peroneal nerve) and Extensor digitorum longus (deep peroneal nerve).
Dissect subcutaneous tissue in plane of skin incision and then dissect between peroneus brevis and EDL to identify fibula and interosseous membrane. Dissect

along interosseous membrane medially to reach lateral surface of tibia.

Dangers: Deep peroneal nerve and anterior tibial artery in anterior compartment. Superficial peroneal nerve, especially where it pierces lateral intermuscular septum.

Medial and lateral approach to ankle fracture:
Discussed in technical station.

Posterior approach lumbar spine for discectomy:
Identify correct level of discectomy with image intensifier, before skin incision (common reason for litigation – wrong level surgery).
Internervous plane: Between erector spinae muscle of both sides. Erector spinae muscle has segmental innervation.
Skin incision - Posterior Midline incision.
Subcutaneous tissue.
Lumbodorsal fascia.
Identify spinous process.
Elevate erector spinae off spinous processes, starting medial and proceed laterally to the facet joints.
Identify ligamentum flavum.
Flavectomy at lamina.
Underlying dura exposed.

Identify intervertebral disc laterally for posterolateral prolapse and perform discectomy, without injuring the dura.

Clinical Knowledge stations

The following questions are collected from previous ST3 interviews. Also look at essential reading section, which will suggest topics to be read. This should cover most of the topics, although one has to be realistic and accept that it is impossible to discuss all orthopaedic clinical scenarios in this interview book.

Q1. You are ST3 on call. You are called at 10PM to see a patient who has right foot drop. Patient underwent right total hip replacement earlier in the day.

Facts – Peroneal division of sciatic nerve more commonly affected than tibial division. Posterior acetabular retractors can cause pressure symptoms on sciatic nerve, posterior acetabular drill holes can cause sciatic nerve injury, cement extrusion from acetabulum can cause thermal injury, post operative haematoma can cause compression injury, excessive lengthening of the leg can cause stretch injury, iatrogenic intraoperative nerve laceration (rare).

Seddon's classification – Neuropraxia, Axonotmesis, Neurotmesis.
Neuropraxia: Nerve bruising. Focal demyelination caused usually by local ischemia. Full recovery

possible. No Wallerian degeneration. No fibrillation on EMG.

Axonotmesis: Axon and myelin sheath disruption. Endoneurium intact. Wallerian degeneration distal end. Fibrillations on EMG. Spontaneous recovery possible.

Neurotmesis: Complete nerve division including endoneurium. Wallerian degeneration distal end. Fibrillations on EMG. No spontaneous recovery. Surgical repair necessary for recovery.

Example Answer:

On arrival to ward, I will discuss with ward staff/doctor to obtain more information about the patient. I will then go through clinical notes to assess any relevant past history, any previous sciatic nerve pathologies, read operation notes to know if it was a primary or revision surgery and also look for any complications mentioned during surgery or if the procedure was more complex than usual.

On arrival at patient's bedside, along with chaperone, I will introduce myself and confirm patient details. I will obtain history from patient including any previous sciatic nerve problems, any leg length discrepancies pre surgery, reason surgery was performed, any co morbidities and drug history especially if patient was on any anticoagulants.

I will next proceed to examination. (Remember - Look, feel, move)
I will Look for limb shortening/lengthening, posture (Limb lengthening: can increase risk of sciatic nerve stretch injury, textbooks quote more than 3cm lengthening significant, but this does not need to be the case. Limb shortening: could indicate dislocation). Also look at hip wound dressing to assess for any blood stained leak or for presence of any massive bruising suggestive of possible haematoma. (Haematoma can still be present in the absence of these features).
Next proceed to feel and will assess sensations at foot. Will assess ankle movements. Also assess distal pulses.

If sensations absent/decreased and foot drop present (peroneal division of sciatic nerve affected), patient has sciatic nerve palsy.

Causes for foot drop immediately post hip replacement:
Iatrogenic sciatic nerve injury (Intraoperative injury, likely secondary to posterior retractors).
Hip haematoma.
Limb lengthening.
Dislocated Hip.

My immediate management plan will be to decrease tension on the sciatic nerve by flexing knee by 20 – 30 degrees under pillow. Make sure there are no tight bandages at the hip region.

If suspecting dislocation, I will organise xray.

At this stage, I will inform the patient's consultant regarding the sciatic nerve palsy and starve the patient from midnight. Unlikely he will need to go to theatre overnight. However, if suspecting haematoma, will need to go to theatre in the morning for possible haematoma evacuation.

Q2. You are the registrar on call. A&E registrar refers a patient with open tibia (Gustillo-Anderson 2 type) fracture. What is your management plan?

Need to be thorough with ATLS for this station. Obtain details from A&E and patient. Use AMPLE (Allergies, Medications,Past history, Last meal, Events leading to fracture) format to obtain a quick history from patient.
Subsequently proceed to perform a primary survey/assess patient using ATLS principles.
A (Airway with cervical spine control) - As the patient is talking, airway is clear. C-Spine will be immobilised. Start oxygen inhalation.
B (Breathing) - Proceed to Breathing and assess for bilateral symmetry of chest movements, tracheal position, percuss and auscultate breath sounds bilaterally. Assuming breathing is fine, proceed to assess circulation.
C (Circulation) – Assess for any obvious sources of bleeding, open wounds. In this scenario patient

has tibial fracture. Other sources of bleeding include chest, abdomen, pelvis, long bones. Examine these sources to make sure, no other source of bleeding other than tibia. Note Pulse and BP. (Can ask interviewer if pulse and BP are satisfactory?). Ask assistant to insert 2 large bore cannula and take blood sample for FBC, U&E, Lactate, cross match 4 units. Also request to perform Arterial Blood Gas. Start hartmanns solution 1 litre in each arm.
Monitor circulatory status by assessing Pulse, BP, Urine output, patient's conscious level.
D (Disability) - Assuming circulation is stable, will proceed to assessment of disability. Will perform AVPU (A – Alert, V – Responds to Verbal stimulus, P – Responds to Pain, U – Unresponsive) and Glasgow coma score. Also assess pupil size and reaction.
E (Exposure) - Then proceed to exposure to look for any obvious injuries, need to prevent hypothermia.

Can be asked by interviewer that patient is tachycardic and hypotensive, what will you do?
Answer – look for sources of bleeding – chest, abdomen, pelvis and long bones. Patient has tibial fracture, however it is important to rule out other sources of bleeding. Quickly examine chest, abdomen, pelvis, other long bones. If no other source of bleeding clinically, likely bleeding from fractured tibia. Check bloods, cross match. Start IV Fluids and monitor response. Catheterise to

monitor urine output, if no perineal bruising. Stop any external sources of bleeding. Ask interviewer if the patient responds to fluid challenge. If responds well (hemodynamically stable) to fluid challenge, then proceed to disability assessment.

If not responding to fluid challenge (unlikely from isolated tibia fracture), will need to make a clinical decision regarding possible source of bleeding. Also need to activate major haemorrhage pathway. If any delay in obtaining blood, request for O negative blood.
If suspecting multiple long bone fractures, need to request xrays in resuscitation. If fractures present, assess for neurological status. Assess response to IV fluids/blood transfusion. If circulation stable, will need early stabilisation. If circulation still compromised, need to consider urgent stabilisation.
If suspecting pelvis fracture, needs urgent AP pelvis xray in resuscitation. If fracture not obvious on xray with pelvic binder, need xray without pelvic binder to assess for any open book type fracture. Need to consider discussing with radiologist for angiographic embolisation, if patient hemodynamically unstable.
If abdomen tender, need to rule out intra abdominal bleeding. Patient can have CT scan if hemodynamically stable. If not stable, FAST (focused assessment with sonography for trauma) scan can be performed by A&E or general surgical team.

Management of Open tibia fracture. Follow this sequence for all open fractures.
Analgesia.
Antibiotics ASAP, ideally within 3 hours (follow local guidelines).
Clean wound with saline/ Saline soaked gauze, if any obvious contamination.
Photograph.
Assess distal neuro vascular status.
Splintage with above knee backslab.
Reassess distal neuro vascular status.
Xray
Inform plastic surgery colleagues, T&O Consultant on call, theatre staff, anesthetist, radiographer.

Treatment – Needs wound debridement and surgical stabilisation with intramedullary nail. Will perform external fixation instead of nail, if facture is very comminuted or in the presence of extensive soft tissue loss. With soft tissue loss, nail can still be performed, as long as plastic surgeons can provide early soft tissue cover, within 3 days. Vacuum foam dressings can be used temporarily while awaiting soft tissue cover.
(Read BOAST 4 guideline on open fracture management)

Classes of Haemorrhagic shock:

Class	1	2	3	4
Blood Loss	<15% (750 ml)	15-30% (750 – 1500ml)	30 – 40% (1500 – 2000 ml)	>40% (>2000ml)
Clinical features	Normal pulse rate, Normal Systolic BP	Tachcardia, Normal Systolic BP, Narrow pulse pressure, Elevated Diastolic pressure, Urine output 20-30ml/hr	Tachcardia (>120beats/min), Low systolic BP, Confusion, Tachypnoea, Urine output <20ml/hr	Tachcardia (>120beats/min), Low systolic BP, Confusion, Tachypnoea, No urine output
Treatment	Nil	IV fluids	RBC, treat cause	RBC (Massive haemorrhage protocol), treat cause

Q3. Xray showing displaced Supracondylar elbow fracture in a 8 year old boy who fell off trampoline. You are the orthopaedic registrar on call and have been called to see him in A&E at 11 PM.

On arrival to A&E, obtain history using AMPLE (Allergies, Medications, Past history, Last meal, Events leading to fracture) format. Inspect arm for elbow swelling, assess radial pulse, capillary refill, sensations in median, ulnar and radial nerve distribution at hand. Also assess for motor function of median, anterior interosseus, ulnar and radial nerves. (Pain can limit motor examination).

Review xray. Interviewer might show an xray. (Need to know gartland classification of distal humerus fractures. Extension type fractures divided into 3 types. Type 1 – undisplaced fracture, type 2 displaced but posterior cortex still intact, type 3 – off ended fracture, posterior cortex disrupted)
Xray shows grade 3 supracondylar fracture.
Initial management is to provide analgesia and apply above elbow back slab for comfort. Reassess neurovascular status post application of back slab and obtain check xray.

Example scenarios:
If the distal limb is well perfused, surgery can wait till next morning. These injuries ideally need to be treated on the same day, if patient arrives at daytime. Discuss with T&O Consultant on call.

Overnight operating is usually not required unless patient has absent radial pulse, clinical signs of impaired perfusion of the hand/digits or evidence of threatened skin viability (BOAST 11 Guideline: Supracondylar fracture of humerus in children).
If there is no radial pulse, but the limb is still well perfused (pink pulseless arm), as per BOAST guidelines, brachial artery exploration is not required. However discuss with vascular team and also inform Consultant on call. Patient requires urgent surgery to reduce fracture displacement and reassessment of Radial pulse and perfusion. If no radial pulse and arm is still well perfused, patient could be monitored in the ward (controversial). Discuss with vascular team.

Essential reading: 2 articles on pink pulseless hand following supracondylar elbow fractures with differing early treatment options.

Blakey CM et al., Ischaemia and the pink pulseless hand complicating supracondylar fractures of the humerus in childhood: long term follow up. JBJS(Br) 2009;91-B:1521-5.

Mangat et al., The 'pulseless pink' hand following supracondylar fractures of the humerus in children:the predictive value of nerve palsy. JBJS(Br) 2009;91-B:1521-5.]

If the limb is ischaemic/not well perfused (pale pulseless arm), immediately discuss with vascular team and inform Consultant on call. Also make arrangements for theatre the same night. Inform theatre co-ordinator, on call anaesthetist, radiographer. Discuss with both patient and parents regarding the need for urgent surgery. This patient requires, fracture reduction and k wire stabilisation followed by reassessment of perfusion. If still not well perfused, will need on table angiogram/brachial artery exploration by vascular team.

Questions relating to surgery:
Describe the fixation method?
Patient supine. GA. Elbow extended. Traction counter traction followed by elbow flexion and simultaneous thumb pressure on the displaced distal fragment in a volar direction, followed by pronation of arm and full flexion. Obtain xrays to check reduction.
Proceed to K wire (2 mm) stabilisation.
Cross k wires (1 medial entry and 1 lateral entry) or 2 lateral k wires.

If the fracture does not reduce closed, consider performing open reduction. This can be performed by medial approach, which is also performed to identify ulnar nerve before inserting medial k wire. Reassess circulation following k wire stabilisation. If the limb is still ischaemic, will need brachial artery exploration by vascular surgeon.

Q4. You are the on call registrar at night. A&E refer a 32 year old male patient with shoulder dislocation after a fall from bike.

Take history with AMPLE format.
Examination – Arm posture, shoulder contour, axillary nerve sensation, radial artery pulse, medial nerve, ulnar nerve and radial nerve function distally.
Xray – need atleast 2 views. AP, Axillary, Scapula Y views.
At this stage consider performing closed reduction if there is no fracture involving the neck or a big hill sachs lesion.
In the presence of undisplaced fracture, one needs to be careful with reduction. As fracture can propagate and displace.
In the presence of large hill sachs lesion, the shoulder could have locked in the dislocated position (locked dislocation) and too much force can cause fracture. In the presence of these scenarios, you can either follow the local guidelines or discuss with consultant on call, as patient might require general anaesthesia for reduction.

Reduction maneuver – number of methods described (traction – counter traction). Need to mention what analgesia and sedation you will use before attempting reduction. For sedation, different hospitals have different guidelines. Some hospitals require either A&E registrar or Anaesthetic registar to provide sedation.

Examiner might say – shoulder not reducible, what next?

Will need reduction under General anaesthetic. So will need to discuss with the On call Consultant, theatre coordinator, anaesthetist, radiographer. The examiner might ask as to whether you are happy to reduce the shoulder on your own and also what approaches you know for the shoulder?

As I am a first year registrar, I will need Consultant to be present in theatre. If the shoulder does not reduce closed, will need open reduction, ideally done at the same setting to avoid a second anaesthetic. I know about approaches to shoulder joint, however will need Consultant presence as I still need practice. I would use deltopectoral approach. (See anatomy section for deltopectoral approach)

Q5: You have been called to A&E to see a patient involved in Road traffic collision car versus lamp post, with a pelvic fracture.

AMPLE - history
ATLS approach

You might be questioned about tachycardia/low blood pressure similar to the scenario described previously. Need to know different classes of shock. Need to know about fluid and blood replacement. Know massive transfusion protocol of your hospital. Interviewer might show xray of pelvis fracture. Need to know about classification.
Remember pelvic ring fractures are different from acetabulum fractures. Pelvic binders usually for pelvic ring fractures. If binder not available, use bedsheet.

Pelvic ring fracture classification –
Young & Burgess classification types –
Anterior posterior compression (APC) injury (3 subtypes)
Lateral compression injury (3 subtypes)
Vertical shear injury

Acetabular fractures – Letournel classification.
Elementary fractures (5 subtypes)
Associated fractures (5 subtypes)

Needs CT scan if patient stable. Ideally CT head to pelvis to identify other injuries. If patient not stable, avoid CT scanner.
Patients can either be -
Good responders – pulse and BP stabilize with fluid/blood.
Transient responders – Pulse and BP stabilize temporarily with fluid/blood. Represents on going blood loss.
Poor responders/non responders – Pulse and BP do not stabilize in spite of fluid and blood challenge. Represents ongoing blood loss.

Transient and Poor responders represent ongoing blood loss. They will require either angiographic embolisation or laparotomy for pelvic packing to stop ongoing blood loss. Discuss with Orthopedic and Invasive Radiology consultants on call. If needing laparotomy, discuss with general surgical team.
If working in a hospital without pelvic team, discuss with the regional pelvic service. However patient has to be stabilised ideally in the local hospital.

Q6: Telephone conversation: Discuss with your Consultant regarding a patient you have seen with open femur fracture in A&E.

Use 'SBAR'protocol (discussed in communication section) when discussing with Consultant about patient.

S – Situation
Introduce yourself, check you are speaking to the correct person, and inform patient details.
B – Background
Reason for patient's attendance to Hospital, mechanism of injury, any past medical history.
A – Assessment
Your assessment of patient. Examination findings. In this scenario, mention ATLS findings. Mention about open fracture, type of open wound. Also mention any relevant patient concerns.
R – Remedy
Mention the treatment you have provided including fluid management, blood tests, wound washout, analgesia, antibiotics, splintage. Also mention that you have informed theatre teams, radiographer, anaesthetists, plastic surgeons regarding this patient.

Need to know all available information about the patient before discussing. The information will be provided in the question. Discuss similar to open fracture protocol mentioned earlier. If pen and paper provided can write down the headings quickly, to remind yourself.

Q7: You are called to see a 40 year old patient involved in RTC with knee dislocation.

History – AMPLE format
Examination - ATLS approach.
Knee dislocation (dashboard injury) – recognize it is an emergency and can be associated with neurovascular injury + multi ligament injury. Atleast 3 out of 4 knee ligaments (ACL, PCL, MCL, LCL) disrupted. 50% associated with vascular injury (popliteal artery) at popliteal fossa as artery tethered proximally at adductor hiatus and distally at soleus arch. Dislocation classified based on the position of tibia.

Knee Examination – Knee posture. Assess (and document) dorsalis pedis and posterior tibial pulses. Assess sensations of deep peroneal, superficial peroneal, tibial nerve distributions.
Plan for immediate knee manipulation with analgesia and sedation in resuscitation department. Once knee reduced, reassess pulses and sensations. Apply above knee backslab in about 20degrees of flexion and check xray. If reduction cannot be maintained consider external fixation in theatre.
If unable to reduce in A&E, needs to be reduced in theatre urgently.

If distal pulses absent but well perfused (controversial) in A&E, discuss with vascular team and inform T&O Consultant on call. Will need urgent knee reduction and reassessment.
If distal pulses absent and NOT perfused in A&E, discuss with vascular team and inform T&O Consultant on call. Patient will require urgent knee reduction and reassessment. Following reduction if distal leg still not perfused, will need on table angiogram/exploration/repair/reconstruction of popliteal artery by vascular team.

Indication for CT angiography varies from practice to practice. Some centres tend to perform CT angiogram if there is no pulse with well perfused leg.
If there is no pulse and distal perfusion is not satisfactory, will need to go to theatre immediately. CT angiogram is not indicated.

A pink pulseless limb should be assumed to have arterial injury. Capillary refill can be misleading (BOAST guideline 6 – Management of arterial injuries associated with fracture and dislocation). Limb must be revascularised as an emergency, as warm ischaemia time greater than 3-4 hrs, can lead to irreversible tissue damage and risk of amputation.

Watch for compartment syndrome. Compartment syndrome can occur in the setting of knee dislocation secondary to muscle injury, arterial injury, revascularisation injury. Usually if revascularisation is performed, fasciotomy is done at the same setting.

Q8: You are called to A&E to see a patient with C6/7 fracture dislocation following RTC, on the first day of your registrar job.

AMPLE History.
ATLS protocol, triple immobilisation of neck – hard collar, blocks on either side of head, tape across forehead and chin. Mention about logroll at end of ATLS to palpate entire spine and also to perform per rectal examination assessing for peri anal sensations, anal tone, any bleeding, high riding prostate in males.

Obtain cervical spine xrays (AP, Lateral, Odontod peg view). AP and lateral should include top of T1 vertebra.
CT scan is preferred these days as it can provide more information. Consider scanning the entire spine, as there is about 20% chance of injury elsewhere in the spine. Also if any concerns with abdomen or pelvis, they can be scanned at the same time or a Trauma CT (head to pelvis) performed. In trauma scenarios, especially in major trauma centres, usually Trauma CT (head to pelvis) is preferred.

Spine fracture classification:

Subaxial cervical spine fracture types – compression, burst, flexion-distraction, facet dislocation, facet fracture.
Thoracolumbar fracture classification - Denis 3 column classification: Anterior, middle, posterior columns

Examine spine – Can use examination guidelines as per ASIA (American Spinal Injury Association) chart to identify a neurological level of deficit. If neurology present needs urgent MRI scan.

If at this stage you are asked about further management, assuming you are the Orthopaedic spine registrar on call, you will inform Consultant about the patient. The patient will need to go to theatre urgently for reduction and stabilization of C6/7 fracture dislocation especially in the setting of neurological deficit.

Absent reflexes and loss of sensations in patients with spinal cord injury can be due to spinal shock.

Spinal shock versus Neurogenic shock

Spinal shock – Absent reflexes, flaccid paralysis, absent sensations below the level of spinal cord injury. Usually lasts 48 hrs. Recovery followed by spasticity, hyperreflexia and clonus. Polysynaptic reflex such as bulbocavernous reflex (squeezing on the glans penis or tugging on an indwelling catheter causes anal sphincter contraction) is the first reflex to appear during recovery.

Neurogenic shock – Hypotension, bradycardia in a patient with spinal cord injury, secondary to loss of sympathetic tone and decreased peripheral vascular resistance. Can also have loss of sensations and loss of reflexes sometimes. Can be life threatening and needs to be differentiated from spinal shock. Treated with vasopressors.

Other types of shock:
Hypovolemc shock /Haemorrhagic shock – Secondary to loss of blood volume, characterized by tachycardia, low blood pressure.

Septic shock – Secondary to infection, characterized by tachycardia, warm peripheries, hypotension refractive to fluid replacement, fever or hypothermia, leukocytosis, sickness.

Cardiogenic shock – secondary to inadequate cardiac output due to cardiac pathology such as Myocardial infarctio, arrythymias, valve pathologies etc.

Anaphylactic shock – severe allergic reaction wth throat, tongue, facial swelling, breathlessness, low blood pressure, rash.

Q9: You are the orthopaedic registrar on call and have been called at 2AM by your SHO about a patient, who underwent tibial nailing earlier that day and has been complaining of excruciating pain.

(Read BOAST guideline 10: Diagnosis and management of compartment syndrome of the limbs)
I will discuss with the SHO about the patient. Check clinical notes to confirm the mechanism of injury, past history, drug history, operation performed, analgesia requirement by the patient. Pain in excess of the ordinary will make me concerned about possible compartment syndrome.
I will then assess patient. Introduce myself to patient. Obtain brief history, especially the degree of pain. Examine leg (Look, Feel, Move). Look for any tense swelling, any tight bandages. Feel for stretch pain, tenderness, sensations and pulses. Check toe movements.

As pain is not settling with analgesia, I will remove any tight bandages and elevate the limb. Will reassess in few minutes. If pain persistent and patient has stretch pain, patient will need urgent fasciotomy. I will find out time of last meal, will discuss with theatre co-ordinator regarding availability of theatre space. Inform anaesthetist. Will discuss with consultant on call regarding my concerns.

(If clinically not convincing of compartment syndrome or if the patient is not conscious, can perform compartment pressure measurements. Record diastolic BP. Record intracompartmental pressure with pressure monitoring device. If the difference between these two, is less than 30mm hg or if the absolute intracompartmental pressure is more than 40 mm hg, it indicates compartment syndrome. Remember, Compartment syndrome is manly a clinical diagnosis in awake patients)

What is compartment syndrome?
Increased pressure within a closed osseofascial compartment leading to muscle, nerve and blood vessel damage.

Aetiology:
Trauma – crush injuries, fractures.
Tight casts, dressings.
Arterial injury.
Bleeding disorders.
Extravasation of IV fluids in arm.
Burns.
Post ischemia swelling/reperfusion.

Pathology:
Bleeding/edema in a closed osseofascial compartment leads to increased interstitial pressure. Leads to Myoneural ischemia. Also leads to occlusion of veins, capillaries followed by

arteries. Remember absence of pulse is a late finding in compartment syndrome.

Clinical features:
Symptom - Pain,Pain and Pain out of proportion.
Signs – Stretch pain followed by paraesthesia. Late findings include absent pulse, paralysis.

Treatment – Fasiotomy.

How do you perform fasciotomy of lower limb?
(More details in anatomy section)
Patient supine.
Tourniquet (may or may not be required, depending on the indication for surgery. Useful to have it on anycase, but don't need to inflate it unless required)
2 incision technique,
Posteromedial incision – decompresses superficial and deep posterior compartments. Incision performed about 2 cm posterior to palpable medial border of tibia.
Anterolateral incision – decompresses anterior and lateral compartments. Incision performed 2 cm anterior to fibula.

Q10. You are the orthopaedic registrar on call, asked to see a 35 year old lady with 2 day history of back pain and difficulty passing urine since morning.

This is a cauda equina scenario. As with any other patient, you will start with history taking (AMPLE), examination (Lumbar spine including per rectal examination), differential diagnosis, investigations (MRI).

Cauda equine syndrome is characterised by one or more of the following features - bowel or bladder dysfunction, saddle anaesthesia, disturbance of sexual function, decreased anal tone. In addition patient will have back pain with or without radiation to one or both limbs
Cauda equna syndrome can be divided further into cauda equine syndrome incomplete (CESI) and Cauda Equna syndrome with retention (CESR).
(Essential reading: An Algorithm for Suspected Cauda Equina Syndrome; Ann R Coll Surg Engl. 2009 May; 91(4): 358–359. NV Todd)

Cauda equina Syndrome incomplete (CESI): Patients have impaired bladder/bowel/peri anal sensation, impaired anal tone. However the bladder is still functioning normally.

Cauda equina syndrome with retention (CESR): Patients have complete paralysis of the bladder

leading to painless retention of urine with overflow incontinence.
In CESR, damage is already done.

Studies have shown patients with CESI need urgent decompression to avoid progression to CESR.

Need to know about cauda equina syndrome – symptoms, signs, investigations, treatment.
Read this article freely available online on Cauda Equna Syndrome:
An Algorithm for Suspected Cauda Equina Syndrome; Ann R Coll Surg Engl. 2009 May; 91(4): 358–359. NV Todd
In brief the above paper suggests the following algorithm:
1. Difficulty passing urine with severe pain and without neurological deficit – Admit, pain relief, MRI following day especially in District general hospital
2. Patients with CESI – Urgent MRI either at DGH or local spinal centre followed by decompression. Ongoing debate whether surgery needs to be done same night or next morning.
3. Patients with CESR – ongoing debate whether MRI and surgery needs to be done same night or next day, depends on surgeon's assessment of literature.

What are 'Red Flags' in patients with back pain?

Red flags indicate need for further investigation.

Red flags:

Age <20 or >55 with NEW onset pain.

IVDU, immunocompromised states, recent significant infection, fever, general malaise.

Weight loss (unexplained).

H/O malignancy.

Rest pain.

Bladder or bowel dysfunction.

Progressive neurological deficit.

Disturbed gait, saddle anaesthesia.

B/L sciatica.

Recent trauma.

Thoracic back pain.

What are 'Yellow Flags' in patients with back pain?

Yellow flags indicate risk of progressing to chronic back pain.

Yellw flags:

Negative attitude – 'Back pain is harmful or severely disabling'.

Pain avoidance behavior.

Depression.

Social or financial problems.

Awaiting compensation.

Essential reading:

BOAST (BOA standards of trauma) guidelines.

Damage control orthopaedics.

Clavicle fractures – classification, management.

Proximal humerus fractures – Neer's classification, management, results of ProFHER trial.

Supracondylar elbow fractures – classification, management.

Distal radius fractures – Management. UK DRAFFT trial results.

Carpal tunnel syndrome – clinical features, investigations, treatment.

Hip fractures – classification, treatment.

Femur shaft and distal fractures – treatment.

Proximal tibia fractures – Schatzker classification, treatment.

Tibia shaft fractures – treatment, complications.

Pilon fractures – classification, treatment (Remember Span, Scan, Plan).

Ankle fracture – classification, treatment.

Also read published articles mentioned throughout clinical stations.

Technical skills station

15 minute station. Will be asked to perform a technical exercise on sawbone. I have included indication and patient position along with the surgical technique. You could be asked about these and therefore useful to know.

Question: Perform DHS on sawbone

Indications for DHS:
Intertrochanteric fractures, excluding reverse oblique. (IM nail preferred for reverse oblique)
Basicervical fractures.
Young patients with Intracapsular fractures (can use cannulated screws).

Equipment required:
Synthes DHS kit (if familiar with any other DHS kit, mention that).

Patient position: (need to mention this, however in the interview you will be provided with sawbone).
Supine on Fracture/Traction table
Bolster in perineal region
Non fractured leg in stirrup
Traction on fractured hip.
Ensure adequate space for image intensifier
Fracture position under image intensifier

Aim for anatomic reduction. Medial and posterior cortices have to be aligned at fracture site, especially.

If satisfactory reduction achieved, start antiseptic preparation and draping with universal drape. However if fracture not reduced, try the following maneuvers:
1. Traction to disimpact fragments, abduction and external rotation. Assess for reduction.
2. Traction to disimpact fragments and internal rotation. Assess for reduction.
3. Leadbetter technique to reduce displaced intracapsular neck of femur fracture –
Flex hip to 90degrees (relax muscles around hip), slight adduction, traction, internal rotation to 45degree (relax Y ligament).
Full flexion and adduction. Slight abduction and full extension while maintain traction and internal rotation.

If unable to obtain a satisfactory reduction, plan for open reduction.
Best results are obtained when fracture is anatomically reduced.
Also ensure neck is not in varus.
Obtain AP and Lateral views. Angle between femoral neck and bolster on lateral xray will provide approximate guide to neck anteversion. This is useful to remember while inserting the guidewire.
DHS plates available with 130 degree – 150 degree angles (plates and angle guides are available in 5

degree increments between 130 – 150 degrees, Synthes). If you are using any other DHS plate in your hospital, know their available neck shaft angles. 130 or 135 degree is the most commonly used plate. Remember the angle guide and plate angle should match.

Skin Incision: Guidewire can be placed on top of the drape overlying anterior skin and AP image taken, to identify centre of femoral neck. About 8 cm skin incision starting just proximal to this point along femoral shaft.
Alternatively, start about 5cm distal to tip of greater trochanter (be careful in short patients) and proceed distally.

Deeper dissection:
Incision through subcutaneous tissue.
Incise fascia lata to the length of skin incision or alternatively make a small incision in fascia lata followed by incision with curved tissue scissors.
Travers self retaining retractors.
Incision in perimysium of vastus lateralis.
2 ways to negotiate vastus lateralis. Vastus split or subvastus. In vastus split, vastus lateralis is split in the line of skin incision along femoral shaft. In subvastus, vastus lateralis muscle is elevated of lateral intermuscular septum and the entire vastus lateralis is retracted superiorly with hohmann retractor. Importantly coagulate any perforators during this step.

Technical steps (Synthes DHS plate):
(Optional step) Use blunt end of guidewire on the anterior surface of femoral head and neck and obtain AP image. Ensure the guidewire is in the centre of the neck on AP view. Angle of this guidewire will also provide an approximate idea regarding the amount of anteversion necessary with inserting the actual guidewire.
Alternatively remember neck anteversion from the initial lateral image (angle between femoral neck and bolster on lateral image).

2.5 mm threaded guide wire is inserted with 135 degree angle guide (some hospitals use 130 degree angle guide and 130 degree plate routinely). Ideal position is central in both AP and lateral views of head and neck. This will provide a satisfactory TIP APEX Distance. Wire should stop at subchondral bone. Avoid penetrating the wire through femoral head.
Measure the wire length. Subtract 10mm to set triple reamer length and also lag screw length.
If guide wire measures less than 75mm, use short barrel triple reamer and short barrel DHS plate.
Triple reamer – it is called triple reamer as it simultaneously drills for lag screw, reams for DHS plate barrel and also reams for countersink at plate barrel junction.
Triple ream to predetermined depth, over the guidewire (Should know how to assemble triple reamer yourself, if not sure go to trauma theatre ASAP to learn). Screen with image intensifier to

avoid wire/reamer penetration through femoral head.

If guidewire is pulled out, method of re-insertion: Push the centering sleeve into the reamed hole and slide an inverted DHS screw
onto the sleeve. The guide wire can now be replaced in the screw to reach its original position.

Tap over the guidewire. Make sure not to penetrate the femoral head.
12.7mm Lag screw of adequate length inserted.
The final position of T handle has to be parallel to femoral shaft.
Check position on image intensifier (AP and lateral).
Remove T handle.
Slide 135 degree DHS plate (usually 4 hole) across the lag screw.
Gentle tap with pusher and mallet on plate.
Remove guidewire.
Fix the plate onto shaft with 4.5mm cortical acrews (3.2mm drill).
Check final position with image intensifier (AP and lateral)
Closure – Perimysium of vastus lateralis (optional), fascia lata, subcutaneous tissue, skin.

Tip Apex distance:

It is the sum of distances from tip of the lag screw to apex of femoral head on AP and Lateral. TAD less than 25mm is considered to decrease the risk of screw cutout.

(Baumgaertner et al., The value of the tip-apex distance in predicting failure of fixation of peritrochanteric fractures of the hip. J Bone Joint Surg Am. 1995 Jul;77(7):1058-64)

How to calculate Tip Apex distance?

Calculate magnification factor = actual diameter of lag screw (12.7)/measured diameter of lag screw (x)

= 12.7/x

Calculate sum of distances from tip of lag screw to apex of femoral head on AP and Lateral xrays. Multiply this value with the magnification factor (12.7/x) to obtain Tip Apex distance.

Small Fragment Set:

Screw diameter	Drill	Tap
Cortical - 3.5mm	2.5mm	3.5 mm, do not require tap if using self tapping screws.
Cancellous – 4mm	2.5mm	Usually do not require tap, 4mm tap if required
Locking – 3.5mm	2.8mm	Usually self tapping

Large Fragment set:

Screw diameter	Drill	Tap
Cortical – 4.5mm	3.2mm	4.5mm
Cancellous – 6.5mm	3.2mm	6.5mm
Locking – 5mm	4.3mm	Usually self tapping

Question: Perform ankle fracture fixation on sawbone.

Will be asked to fix ankle fracture on saw bone.
Know screw diameters for small and large fragment sets.
Decide before starting if fracture configuration requires lag screw application.
If applying lag screw, one third tubular plate will act as neutralisation plate.
If lag screw not possible, apply dynamic compression plate – this will provide anatomic reduction by compression and act as a compression plate.

Indications:
Isolated lateral malleolus fractures with talar displacement.
Weber C lateral malleolus fractures (need syndesmotic screw).
Bimalleolar fractures.
Trimalleolar fractures.
Open fractures.

Equipment required:
Small fragment set.
One third tubular plate for lateral malleolus.
Dynamic Compression plate, if fracture configuration does not permit lag screw.
For medial malleolus, either partially threaded cancellous screws or tension band wire depending upon size of the fragment. For this example, medial

malleolus fragment is large enough to accept 2 partially threaded cancellous screws.

Patient position:
Supine with tourniquet. Sandbag under ipsilateral buttock to rotate leg internally for lateral malleolus fracture fixation. Fractured ankle on rectangle block/bolster. Obtain image intensifier images to ensure adequate images possible.

Procedure: (Assuming weber B oblique lateral malleolus and transverse fracture medial malleolus).

Antiseptic Preparation till tourniquet. Drape till tourniquet.

Lateral malleolus:
Skin - Lateral incision at distal fibula, in mid fibular plane.
Dissect subcutaneous tissue in line with skin incision, along mid fibular plane.
Remember, Superficial peroneal nerve lies anterior and sural nerve posterior to fibula.
Identify fibula fracture.
Clear fracture site by elevating soft tissues around fracture with periosteal elevator.
Keep soft tissue dissection to minimal to preserve blood supply.
Reduce fracture with pointed reduction forceps.
Apply lag screw. – drill proximal cortex with 3.5mm drill. Insert drill sleeve and drill distal cortex with

2.5mm drill. Measure and Insert 3.5mm fully threaded cortical screw.
Asses reduction on xrays.

Apply one third tubular plate (neutralization plate). Length of the plate to be decided based on fracture position and length. Ideally require 6 cortices proximally (3 cortical screws) and 3 cancellous screws distally.
Clamp plate to bone. Drill with 2.5mm drill. Use fully threaded 3.5mm cortical screws proximal fibula(cortical bone) and fully threaded 4mm cancellous screws at the lateral malleolus (cancellous bone). Will require 3.5mm tap prior to inserting cortical screws, if the screws are not self-tapping.
Assess reduction on theatre xrays.

Check for syndesmosis by external rotation stress test or hook test.

Medial malleolus:
Curved skin incision at fracture site. (curve anteriorly as tendons and neurovascular bundle lie posterior to medial malleolus).
Incise subcutaneous tissue in same plane.
Identify fracture site.
Clear fracture site.
Reduce fracture with pointed reduction forceps.
(Optional)Insert 2mm k wire to keep fracture reduced.
Check reduction under image intensifier.

2.5mm drill, measure, apply 4mm partially threaded cancellous screws with or without washer.
Repeat similar step and apply second screw.
Do not penetrate the joint.
Check xray.

Closure –
Subcutaneous tissue 2-0 vicryl and subcuticular monocryl.
Below knee backslab.

Post op instructions:
Foot elevation.
Change backslab to below knee non weight bearing cast tomorrow.
Cast for 2 or 6 weeks (depending on fracture stability).
Non weight bearing 6 weeks.
Clinic 2 weeks for wound check and check xray.

What is lag screw?
Lag screw provides compression across fracture. Lag screw only engages in the bone distal to fracture. The proximal cortex acts as a gliding hole. As the screw tightens, distal bone which is held by the screw is compressed against the proximal bone which is held by the screw head. Lag screw needs to be applied perpendicular to the fracture to provide effective compression.

Question: Perform Tension Band wire fixation on sawbone olecranon fracture.

Indication:
Displaced transverse Olecranon fracture proximal to level of coronoid, without communition.

Equipment:
2 x 2mm k wires.
Tension band wire set.
18G wire.

Patient position:
Lateral position – Arm on stirrup.
Supine position – Arm across chest.
Ensure adequate imaging is possible.

Procedure:
Arm Tourniquet.
Antiseptic preparation and draping to tourniquet level.
Skin incision – posterior midline approach. Linear incision with curve radially around the olecranon tip, to avoid wound across olecranon tip.
Dissect subcutaneous tissue in sae plane.
Identify olecranon fracture.
Reduce fracture with pointed reduction forceps.
Apply 2 x 2mm k wires.
Ensure wires not intraarticular.
Also ensure wires are stopped just anterior to the anterior ulna cortex.
Check position with image intensifier.

2mm drill hole transversely at distal fragment 4 cm distal to fracture.
Pass 18G wire across ulna transverse hole.
Loop it taking across (superiorly) both k wires and bring it back to join the starting wire in figure of 8 fashion.
Wires should cross at fracture site.
Wires can be tensioned on one side or on both sides.
Tensioning is a combination of pulling and twisting.
Check position under image intensifier.
Back out k wires by 5 mm.
Cut K wire about 2 cm protruding.
Bend wires
Make a small longitudinal split in the triceps tendon.
With a small punch and toffee mallet both wires are pushed forward to bury the k wires.

Closure:
Subcutaneous 2-0 viryl.
Subcuticular 3-0 monocryl.
Mepore dressing.
Wool and crepe dressing.

Post operative instructions:
Mobilise as tolerated.
Reduce dressings after 48 hrs.
Wound check and check xray at 2 weeks.

Principle of tension band wire fixation: Tension on the non articular side is converted to compression at the articular side. Hence it is important to start early range of movements.

Question: Perform Intercostal drain (chest drain)on mannequin (Not been asked before).

Tension pneumothorax (first line treatment is needle decompression)
Ventilated patient with pneumothorax.
Traumatic pneumothorax/Haemothorax

Most common reason orthopaedic surgeon gets involved is in trauma situation.

Equipment: chest drain kit (usually available in A&E)
To drain traumatic pneumothorax/haemothorax, chest drain size 26ch and above.
To drain spontaneous pneumothorax, chest drain size12ch.

Patient position:
Patient either at 45degree inclination from supine or sitting up in a forward lean position. Arm raised over head to expose axillary region.

Antiseptic preparation to skin.

Local anaesthesia infiltration:

10 ml of 1% lignocaine in skin and through the layers of the chest wall in the direction of chest tube.

Incision :

5th intercostal space, mid axillary line. (Rib spaces are counted down from the 2nd rib at the sternomanubrial joint).

Identify upper border of lower rib.

Transverse incision at upper border of lower rib (neurovascular bundle at lower border of rib)

Controlled spreading of subcutaneous tissues and muscles. A curved clamp can be used for blunt dissection. Once pleura is reached, it is penetrated with the blunt curved clamp. The entry is confirmed by gush of air/blood.

Chest drain is inserted and connected to underwater seal. Chest drain should be inserted so that the last hole of the drain is inside the thoracic cavity. However if passed too far into the chest, drains can cause severe intractable pain as they abut the mediastinum.

The drain is secured with sutures to skin.

Underwater seal for the drain: It is always kept below the level of the patient to allow air to escape through the drain but not to re-enter the thoracic cavity. With respiration, water column in the chest drain tube will swing up and down.

Obtain chest xray to confirm position.

Questions Index